Neurogenesis and Brain Development - Advances and Challenges

Edited by Xinhua Zhang

Published in London, United Kingdom

Neurogenesis and Brain Development - Advances and Challenges
http://dx.doi.org/10.5772/intechopen.1008612
Edited by Xinhua Zhang

Contributors
Alvaro Duque, Emma Burke, Farjana Yasmin, Francisco J. Ocaranza, Gang Mai, Guanting Lu, Janny Piñeiro-Llanes, Juan C. Sáez, Lucy Greene, Masahito Nakazaki, Pasko Rakic, Phil Barello, Qiongling Peng, Rodrigo Cristofoletti, Valeria Mendoza-Silva, Xiao Liu, Yury M. Morozov

First published in London, United Kingdom, 2026 by IntechOpen

IntechOpen is the global imprint of INTECHOPEN LIMITED, registered in England and Wales, registration number: 11086078, 167-169 Great Portland Street, London, W1W 5PF, United Kingdom

For EU product safety concerns: IN TECH d.o.o., Prolaz Marije Krucifikse Kozulić 3, 51000 Rijeka, Croatia, info@intechopen.com or visit our website at intechopen.com.

British Library Cataloguing-in-Publication Data
A catalogue record for this book is available from the British Library

Neurogenesis and Brain Development - Advances and Challenges
Edited by Xinhua Zhang
p. cm.
Print ISBN 978-1-83634-638-8
Online ISBN 978-1-83634-637-1
eBook (PDF) ISBN 978-1-83634-639-5

Meet the editor

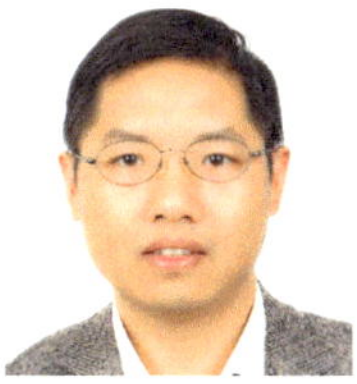

Professor Xinhua Zhang, born in 1971, holds a Ph.D. and is a distinguished Teaching Master in Jiangsu Province, leading national and provincial first-class undergraduate and excellent courses. He is a standing committee member of the Chinese Society of Sports Anatomy and a council member of the Jiangsu Society for Neuroscience and the Jiangsu Anatomical Society. He has been honored as an outstanding young teacher in Jiangsu's "Qinglan Project" and as a scientific leader in the "333 Project". Professor Zhang has completed multiple teaching and research projects and has published in top journals such as Nature. He was an academic editor for "Hippocampus." His research has garnered several prestigious awards, including the Natural Science Award from the Ministry of Education and several provincial science and technology awards.

Contents

Preface **IX**

Section 1
Neural Regeneration **1**

Chapter 1 **3**
From Stem Cells to Vesicles: A Comprehensive Review of MSC and MSC-EV Therapeutics for Spinal Cord Injury
by Masahito Nakazaki

Chapter 2 **25**
Regenerative Therapy for Ischemic Brain Injury Using Neural Stem Cells: Mechanisms, Enhancement, and Impact on Neurogenesis
by Xiao Liu

Section 2
Brain Development **45**

Chapter 3 **47**
Microphysiological Systems: Advancing Insights into Brain Development and Disorders
by Farjana Yasmin, Rodrigo Cristofoletti and Janny Piñeiro-Llanes

Chapter 4 **75**
Molecular Analysis of Chinese FOXG1-Related Encephalopathy
by Guanting Lu, Gang Mai and Qiongling Peng

Chapter 5 **101**
Perspective Chapter: From Embryonic Archives to Translational Insights – Reusing Nonhuman Primate Brain Data to Decode Development and Reduce Animal Sacrifice
by Alvaro Duque, Phil Barello, Lucy Greene, Emma Burke, Valeria Mendoza-Silva, Yury M. Morozov and Pasko Rakic

Chapter 6 **121**
The Impact of Hemichannel-Mediated Neuroinflammation at Early Stages of CNS Ontogeny in the Development of Adult Neuropsychiatric Diseases
by Francisco J. Ocaranza and Juan C. Sáez

Preface

The human brain is one of the most intricate systems in nature, and the mechanisms underlying its development and regeneration remain a central focus of neuroscience research. Nonetheless, injuries and diseases affecting the nervous system, such as stroke, spinal cord injury, neurodegenerative disorders, and neurodevelopmental conditions, impose a significant burden on hundreds of millions of patients and their families worldwide. Conventional therapeutic strategies often offer symptomatic relief but seldom achieve fundamental restoration of neural structure and function. In this context, elucidating the intrinsic principles of brain development and leveraging the brain's inherent regenerative capacity have emerged as crucial aspirations for overcoming current therapeutic limitations and transforming the paradigm for treating neurological disorders. This book systematically synthesizes key advancements in this rapidly evolving field, bridges the gap between basic research and clinical application, and provides a comprehensive roadmap for future researchers.

This volume compiles insights from prominent research teams worldwide, offering a comprehensive, interdisciplinary knowledge framework encompassing central and peripheral neurogenesis, mechanisms of brain development, and related disease models. In Section I, the focus is directed towards the cutting-edge field of "Neural Regeneration". The initial chapter explores the intricate interaction between adult neurogenesis and neuroplasticity, underscoring their essential roles in brain repair and the preservation of cognitive function. Following this, the book employs spinal cord injury as a model to systematically examine how therapies utilizing mesenchymal stem cells and their derived extracellular vesicles facilitate functional recovery. This is achieved through mechanisms such as the repair of the blood-spinal cord barrier, immune modulation, and neuroprotection. The text vividly illustrates the paradigm shift in therapeutic strategies from traditional "cell transplantation" to innovative "cell-free vesicle" applications. In addressing ischemic brain injury, the book further elaborates on the significant potential of neural stem cell therapy and emphasizes novel bioengineering approaches, such as metabolic glycoengineering. These strategies notably enhance stem cell survival, migration, and integration by altering cell surface properties, thereby optimizing therapeutic outcomes. In Section II, our focus shifts to the enigmatic processes and modeling of "Brain Development". This section of the book elucidates critical milestones in brain development, spanning from embryogenesis to adulthood, and highlights the transformative technology of cerebral organoids. These in vitro cultivated "mini-brains" offer valuable insights into normal developmental processes and serve as potent platforms for modeling intricate neurodevelopmental and neurodegenerative disorders, including Down syndrome, autism spectrum disorder, and Alzheimer's disease. Simultaneously, the book delves into the molecular mechanisms underlying specific developmental disorders, including the genetic analysis of FOXG1-related encephalopathy, thereby laying a foundation for accurate diagnosis and prospective gene therapies.

Additionally, it investigates the enduring effects of early-life neuroinflammation, facilitated by mechanisms such as connexin hemichannels, on brain architecture, providing a novel perspective on the developmental origins of adult neuropsychiatric disorders. The book emphasizes the essential roles of technological innovation and resource integration in advancing the field. For example, the endocannabinoid system, functioning as a crucial neuromodulatory mechanism, regulates activity in brain regions such as the olfactory bulb, thereby offering novel therapeutic targets for conditions like epilepsy and schizophrenia. Concurrently, the initiative to develop standardized datasets on embryonic brain development in non-human primates promotes the sharing and reutilization of scientific resources. This approach is not only an ethical obligation to improve research reproducibility but also a critical strategy for expediting scientific discovery.

Despite the promising prospects, significant challenges persist. The safety and long-term efficacy of stem cell therapies, the functional maturity and standardization of organoids, the heterogeneity of complex disorders, and the accompanying ethical considerations constitute substantial obstacles to the translation of research into clinical application. Future advancements will undoubtedly depend on enhanced interdisciplinary collaboration, integrating cutting-edge technologies such as single-cell sequencing, gene editing, microfluidic chips, and artificial intelligence. These technologies will be crucial for the precise decoding and manipulation of neurogenesis and brain development at the molecular, cellular, and systems levels. By elucidating the fundamental principles of brain construction and remodeling, we anticipate the development of effective strategies to promote neural regeneration, repair damaged circuits, and potentially reverse neurodegenerative processes.

This book aims to serve as a comprehensive reference for researchers, clinicians, and graduate students in neuroscience, regenerative medicine, developmental biology, and related disciplines, providing both foundational theories and forward-looking perspectives. We assert that each advancement in understanding the mechanisms underlying brain formation and repair constitutes a significant step towards the eventual conquest of neurological diseases. We hope that this book will inspire novel ideas, illuminate new avenues of exploration, and contribute to a promising future for the field of neuroscience.

Xinhua Zhang
Department of Human Anatomy,
Co-Innovation Center of Neuroregeneration,
Nantong University,
Nantong, China

Section 1

Neural Regeneration

Chapter 1

From Stem Cells to Vesicles: A Comprehensive Review of MSC and MSC-EV Therapeutics for Spinal Cord Injury

Masahito Nakazaki

Abstract

Spinal cord injury (SCI) remains a devastating neurological condition with limited therapeutic options, presenting a significant unmet medical need. This review examines the evolving landscape of mesenchymal stem/stromal cell (MSC) and MSC-derived extracellular vesicle (MSC-EV) therapies for SCI treatment. We explore the biological properties of MSCs, including their immunomodulatory capacity and secretome, and evaluate preclinical evidence demonstrating their efficacy in promoting functional recovery through blood-spinal cord barrier repair, neuroprotection, and immunomodulation. The review highlights the paradigm shift from cellular to vesicular approaches, with MSC-EVs emerging as promising cell-free alternatives that maintain therapeutic benefits while offering advantages in safety, storage, and targeted delivery. Clinical translation progress is assessed, including outcomes from recent trials showing safety and potential efficacy of MSC therapies in human SCI patients. Despite promising results, significant challenges remain in standardization, potency testing, and manufacturing of MSC-EV therapies. Future research should focus on optimizing isolation protocols, enhancing potency assays, and identifying specific EV subpopulations with targeted therapeutic effects. This review provides critical insights into current knowledge and future directions for developing these regenerative approaches to improve SCI patient outcomes.

Keywords: spinal cord injury, mesenchymal stem/stromal cells, extracellular vesicles, neural plasticity, exosomes

1. Introduction

1.1 Overview of spinal cord injury

Traumatic spinal cord injury (SCI) is a devastating neurological condition with profound medical and socioeconomic consequences, affecting millions globally and predominantly impacting young adults [1]. Beyond the substantial lifetime economic burden, SCI drastically curtails quality of life, often resulting in paralysis, sensory deficits, and autonomic dysfunction, thereby underscoring the urgent need for effective therapeutic strategies [2].

The pathophysiology of SCI involves an immediate primary mechanical insult, followed by a prolonged secondary injury cascade characterized by inflammation and vascular disruption, critically including the breakdown of the blood-spinal cord barrier (BSCB) [3, 4]. The primary injury results from the initial physical trauma, causing immediate tissue damage and neuronal death. The secondary injury cascade, evolving over hours to weeks, encompasses multiple pathological processes including ischemia, excitotoxicity, oxidative stress, inflammation, and apoptosis, significantly expanding the lesion and limiting functional recovery [4].

Persistent BSCB compromise is a critical component of this secondary injury process. The BSCB, a specialized vascular interface that maintains spinal cord homeostasis, becomes severely compromised following SCI, leading to increased permeability and infiltration of inflammatory cells and cytotoxic molecules into the spinal cord parenchyma [4, 5]. This barrier dysfunction allows inflammatory cell infiltration and exacerbates tissue damage, significantly limiting functional recovery and highlighting the BSCB as a key therapeutic target [6].

1.2 Current treatment limitations

Current therapeutic options for SCI, primarily surgical stabilization and rehabilitation, offer limited functional restoration and do not address the underlying neural damage [7]. Surgical interventions aim to decompress the spinal cord and stabilize the spine, while rehabilitation focuses on maximizing remaining function and preventing complications. However, neither approach directly promotes neural repair or regeneration.

The intrinsic regenerative capacity of the central nervous system is notably restricted, compounded by an inhibitory environment at the lesion site, characterized by glial scarring and myelin-associated inhibitors that impede axonal regrowth [8, 9]. The glial scar, while initially protective by containing inflammation, ultimately creates a physical and chemical barrier to axonal regeneration. Myelin-associated inhibitors like Nogo, myelin-associated glycoprotein (MAG), and oligodendrocyte-myelin glycoprotein (OMgp) further impede axonal growth.

Consequently, individuals with SCI, especially those with complete injuries, face limited prospects for significant neurological improvement. This therapeutic deficit has spurred intensive research into regenerative strategies, with cell-based therapies emerging as a particularly promising avenue.

1.3 Emergence of cell-based therapies

Mesenchymal stem/stromal cells (MSCs) have garnered significant attention for SCI treatment, primarily due to their immunomodulatory properties and secretion of trophic factors, rather than direct cell replacement [10, 11]. The therapeutic paradigm has evolved from initial expectations of cell replacement to recognition of paracrine effects as the predominant mechanism of action.

Intravenously administered MSCs exert therapeutic effects via paracrine mechanisms, releasing a complex secretome of growth factors, cytokines, and extracellular vesicles (EVs) that collectively promote neuroprotection, modulate inflammation, and stabilize the BSCB [12–15]. This secretome influences multiple aspects of the injury response, including immunomodulation, neuroprotection, angiogenesis, and tissue repair.

More recently, attention has shifted toward MSC-derived EVs as a cell-free therapeutic alternative, offering potential advantages in safety and targeted delivery. It was demonstrated that MSC-EVs specifically target M2-type macrophages at the SCI site, highlighting their potential for selective immunomodulation [16]. Furthermore, studies have shown that MSC-derived EVs carrying specific cargo can promote neurological function recovery in SCI models through mechanisms such as enhancing neuronal autophagy [17].

This evolution from cellular to vesicular therapeutic approaches represents a paradigm shift in regenerative medicine for SCI, potentially offering more refined, safer, and more accessible treatment options. This review examines the biological properties and therapeutic potential of MSCs and MSC-EVs for SCI, with particular focus on their mechanisms of action, preclinical and emerging clinical evidence, and challenges for clinical translation.

2. Mesenchymal stem/stromal cells (MSCs)

2.1 Biological properties and therapeutic potential

Mesenchymal stem/stromal cells (MSCs) are multipotent cells identified by plastic adherence, specific surface antigen expression (CD73+, CD90+, CD105+; CD34-, CD45-, CD14- or CD11b-, CD79α- or CD19-, HLA-DR-), and *in vitro* trilineage differentiation potential into osteoblasts, adipocytes, and chondrocytes [18, 19]. These defining characteristics, established by the International Society for Cell & Gene Therapy, provide standardized criteria for MSC identification across research studies. Initially identified in bone marrow, MSCs have since been isolated from diverse sources including adipose tissue, umbilical cord, dental pulp, and other tissues, each exhibiting subtle differences in therapeutic potency [20]. Bone marrow-derived MSCs (BM-MSCs) remain the most extensively studied, though umbilical cord-derived MSCs (UC-MSCs) have gained attention for their greater proliferative capacity and potentially enhanced immunomodulatory properties. Culture expansion methods, such as using autologous serum, significantly influence MSC proliferation and stability, a technique translated to clinical applications for neurological injuries [21–23].

A cardinal therapeutic attribute of MSCs is their profound immunomodulatory capacity, crucial for mitigating destructive inflammation in neurological injuries [24]. MSCs influence both innate and adaptive immunity through cell contact and secretion of factors like prostaglandin E2 (PGE2) and transforming growth factor-beta (TGF-β) [25]. They promote the polarization of macrophages from a pro-inflammatory M1 to an anti-inflammatory M2 phenotype, a shift correlated with functional recovery in SCI models [14, 15]. Furthermore, MSCs inhibit T-cell proliferation and modulate their differentiation toward regulatory phenotypes, contributing to a microenvironment conducive to tissue repair [26].

The therapeutic benefits of MSCs are now largely attributed to their secretome, a complex milieu of soluble factors and EVs exerting paracrine effects [27]. This includes neurotrophic factors like brain-derived neurotrophic factor (BDNF), angiogenic factors such as vascular endothelial growth factor (VEGF), and EVs carrying proteins and microRNAs [28]. BDNF-hypersecreting MSCs, for instance, enhanced corticospinal tract sprouting and neuronal preservation in SCI models [29].

MSC-secreted factors also accelerate BSCB restoration, a critical mechanism for their therapeutic efficacy in SCI [6, 14].

The rationale for MSC application in SCI encompasses their multifaceted properties addressing several pathological aspects of injury. They modulate the hostile inflammatory environment by shifting macrophage polarization, as shown in studies where MSCs increased the M2/M1 macrophage ratio in SCI lesions [14, 15]. Neurotrophic factors from MSCs protect neurons and promote axonal growth and neural plasticity [30]. The compromised vasculature and BSCB dysfunction are also targeted; MSC infusion accelerates BSCB repair, reducing edema and inflammatory infiltration [6, 14]. Practical advantages include ease of isolation, expansion, cryopreservation, good safety profiles, and the potential for autologous use [21, 22]. These attributes underpin the extensive investigation of MSCs for SCI (**Figure 1**).

2.2 Evidence in rodent models

Rodent contusion models, mimicking human SCI biomechanics and BSCB disruption, have been pivotal in preclinical MSC evaluation [4, 6]. Contusion injuries, often induced by impactors such as the Infinite Horizon impactor, create complex pathology similar to human SCI, including primary mechanical damage and subsequent secondary injury cascades [14]. For instance, several studies employed a 22.5 Newton impact at the T9 level in adult male Sprague-Dawley rats to create severe contusive SCI [14, 15, 31].

Intravenous MSC administration in these models consistently improves locomotor function, assessed by scales like the Basso-Beattie-Bresnahan (BBB) score [32]. It was demonstrated that intravenous infusion of MSCs 1 week after contusive SCI significantly improved BBB scores compared to vehicle-treated controls, with improvements beginning within the first week post-infusion and persisting throughout the

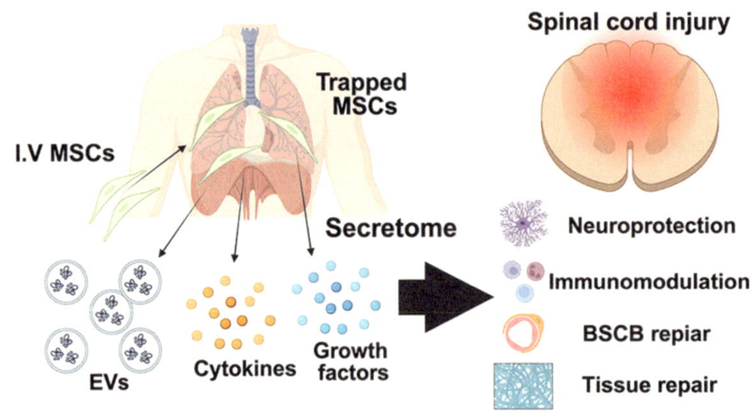

Figure 1.
Therapeutic mechanisms of Mesenchymal Stem/Stromal Cells (MSCs) in spinal cord injury repair. The figure illustrates the proposed mechanisms by which MSCs contribute to spinal cord injury repair. Intravenously administered MSCs (I.V MSCs, left) migrate toward the injury site, though many become trapped in the lungs and other organs (Trapped MSCs, upper right). Both populations of MSCs secrete a complex array of bioactive molecules collectively known as the secretome. The secretome consists primarily of extracellular vesicles (EVs), cytokines, and growth factors. These secreted factors mediate multiple therapeutic effects at the injury site (right), including neuroprotection of remaining neural tissue, immunomodulation to reduce inflammatory damage, blood-spinal cord barrier (BSCB) repair to restore vascular integrity, and promotion of tissue repair through enhanced cellular regeneration and extracellular matrix remodeling. This paracrine mechanism suggests that MSC-derived therapeutic effects may be achievable even when direct cell engraftment at the injury site is limited.

observation period [33]. These functional improvements are often correlated with accelerated BSCB repair, characterized by reduced vascular permeability and upregulation of tight junction proteins (e.g., ZO-1, occludin) shortly after MSC infusion, suggesting a primary role for secreted factors [6, 14].

MSCs exert neuroprotective effects by reducing neuronal and oligodendrocyte apoptosis and fostering an M2 macrophage-dominant microenvironment, which diminishes pro-inflammatory cytokine levels [14, 34]. MSC transplantation after SCI has been shown to increase the proportion of M2 macrophages at the lesion site, correlating with improved functional recovery [34]. Secreted neurotrophic factors like BDNF further contribute to neuronal survival and axonal growth [29]. It was reported that MSCs, particularly those engineered to overexpress BDNF, significantly increased axonal sprouting and corticospinal tract protection in a rat SCI model [29].

While intravenous infusion is clinically translatable, it results in limited MSC engraftment at the SCI site, with cells primarily localizing to the lungs [6]. Despite this, significant functional benefits are observed, strongly indicating that MSCs act via secreted factors, particularly EVs, which can cross the compromised BSCB and interact with target cells, such as M2 macrophages, within the lesion [14, 16]. This paracrine action through EVs is increasingly recognized as the dominant mode of MSC therapeutic efficacy in SCI, discussed in the next section.

Studies demonstrated that even in chronic SCI, MSC infusion significantly reduced BSCB permeability and improved functional outcomes, suggesting the therapeutic window for vascular repair extends beyond the acute injury phase [35, 36]. Further studies revealed that intravenous MSC infusion alters gene expression in the motor cortex of rats with SCI, identifying differentially expressed genes in motor cortices after MSC infusion compared to vehicle controls [37]. This suggests MSCs can trigger remote gene expression responses in the brain, potentially activating regenerative pathways and enhancing neural connectivity.

The consistent observation of BSCB stabilization, immunomodulation, and associated functional benefits across multiple studies underscores key therapeutic mechanisms of MSCs in SCI and provides robust preclinical evidence supporting their clinical translation.

2.3 MSCs and neural plasticity: Mechanisms of circuit reorganization

Beyond their immunomodulatory and neuroprotective effects, MSCs play crucial roles in promoting neural plasticity and circuit reorganization following SCI. Recent evidence suggests that MSCs can facilitate the formation of novel neural pathways and enhance existing connections through multiple mechanisms.

A groundbreaking study demonstrated that intravenously infused MSCs promote the formation of enhanced axonal networks in corticospinal tracts (CSTs) after SCI [38]. The study revealed bridging communications between the dorsal CST and axons in the lateral funiculus just above and below the lesion core, suggesting either axonal regeneration or enhancement of pre-existing fine caliber axon collaterals. The authors proposed that MSCs activate a compensatory system in the injured nervous system by enhancing axonal diameter and conduction velocity, potentially through synaptic reorganization.

MSCs promote neural plasticity through secretion of key neurotrophic factors. BDNF-hypersecreting MSCs have been shown to significantly enhance corticospinal tract sprouting and protection [29]. The BDNF-TrkB signaling cascade activated by MSC-secreted BDNF promotes dendritic spine formation, synaptic maturation, and long-term potentiation—fundamental processes for neural plasticity [39].

MSCs facilitate synaptic remodeling through multiple pathways. They upregulate synaptic proteins including synaptophysin and PSD-95 and GAP-43, markers associated with active synaptogenesis [40]. Additionally, MSCs modulate the expression of guidance molecules such as semaphorins and ephrins, which direct appropriate synaptic connections during circuit reconstruction [41].

The functional significance of MSC-induced plasticity is evidenced by electrophysiological studies showing enhanced synaptic transmission and improved neural conduction in MSC-treated SCI animals [42]. MSCs promote the formation of functional synapses by increasing the expression of vesicular transporters and neurotransmitter receptors at newly formed connections [43].

Collectively, these findings demonstrate that MSCs orchestrate a comprehensive program of neural plasticity following SCI, from structural enhancement of corticospinal networks to molecular regulation of synaptic function. This multifaceted approach to promoting plasticity—combining trophic support, gene expression modulation, and direct synaptic remodeling—underlies the functional improvements observed in MSC-treated animals and provides a mechanistic foundation for understanding how their secreted factors, particularly EVs, mediate therapeutic effects.

3. MSC-derived extracellular vesicles (MSC-EVs)

3.1 MSC-EV play a vital role in the therapeutic mechanism of MSC therapy

The therapeutic paradigm for MSCs has evolved significantly, with growing evidence indicating that EVs are key mediators of MSC efficacy. The “paracrine hypothesis” posits that MSCs exert beneficial effects largely through secreted bioactive molecules, including EVs, rather than direct cell replacement (**Figure 1**) [6, 14, 24, 27]. This represents a fundamental shift in understanding, positioning MSC-EVs as central effectors in MSC therapy.

Compelling evidence for this paradigm in SCI treatment has been provided, demonstrating that fractionated intravenous administration of MSC-derived small EVs (sEVs) mimicked the therapeutic effects of a single MSC infusion [14]. Both treatments yielded comparable improvements in locomotor recovery, increased M2 macrophage polarization, upregulated transforming growth factor-beta (TGF-β), enhanced expression of tight junction proteins, and reduced BSCB permeability [14]. This functional equivalence suggests that MSC-sEVs can recapitulate major therapeutic benefits of their parent cells.

The observation that intravenously delivered MSCs primarily lodge in the lungs yet produce therapeutic effects in distant organs like the spinal cord further supports the role of EVs as mediators of MSC action [6, 16]. It has been demonstrated that MSCs trapped in the lungs after intravenous administration are activated to secrete anti-inflammatory factors, including EVs, which then reach distant injury sites [44]. This model of “activated MSCs” as systemic factories of therapeutic EVs explains how limited cell engraftment can produce widespread benefits.

MSC-EVs appear to regulate gene expression and protein production in target cells through their RNA and protein cargo. For instance, miR-21 carried by MSC-EVs can downregulate pro-apoptotic genes and promote axonal growth [45], while miR-146a modulates inflammatory pathways [46]. The ability of EVs to transfer functional RNAs and proteins that influence cell behavior represents a powerful mechanism for tissue repair and regeneration.

The central role of EVs in MSC therapy has profound implications for therapeutic development, suggesting that EV-based approaches might offer a refined alternative to whole-cell treatments while maintaining equivalent efficacy.

3.2 Characterization and advantages

According to Minimal information for studies of extracellular vesicles (MISEV 2023), EVs are defined as particles released from cells, delimited by a lipid bilayer, and unable to replicate on their own (i.e., they do not contain a functional nucleus) [47]. This updated definition removed the term "naturally released" from the MISEV2018 definition to avoid unintended exclusion of engineered EVs or those produced under various culture conditions. Small EVs (sEVs, 30–150 nm), often previously called exosomes, form through the invagination of multivesicular body (MVB) membranes, creating intraluminal vesicles (ILVs) that are released upon MVB fusion with the plasma membrane. Larger EVs, such as those previously termed microvesicles (100–1000 nm), form through direct budding from the plasma membrane. Together, these heterogeneous vesicle populations constitute the EV fraction of the MSC secretome.

Rather than using terms associated with biogenesis pathways that are difficult to establish (such as "exosomes" or "microvesicles"), MISEV2023 recommends operational extensions to the term "EV" based on physical characteristics (size, density), biochemical composition (surface markers like CD63+/CD81+), or descriptions of cell origin (MSC-derived EVs) and conditions of production. This nomenclature shift reflects the field's recognition that definitive characterization of biogenesis-based subtypes is challenging, with no universal molecular markers for specific EV subtypes.

MSC-EVs offer significant advantages over cellular therapies for SCI [26]. They present a minimal risk of tumorigenicity and uncontrolled proliferation, a critical safety consideration for CNS applications [48]. MSC-EVs also demonstrate an enhanced ability to cross the BSCB compared to whole cells; observations indicated that labeled MSC-EVs trafficked to SCI sites, unlike parent MSCs that lodge in the lungs [6, 14, 16]. This selective biodistribution enhances therapeutic delivery. Furthermore, MSC-EVs offer practical benefits in manufacturing, extended storage stability at −80°C, and the potential for repeated administration without immune rejection [49, 50].

3.3 Preclinical evidence in SCI

Preclinical evaluation of MSC-EVs for SCI predominantly utilizes rodent models, particularly rats, due to their well-characterized injury responses and the availability of standardized injury paradigms [14, 15]. Study designs typically involve inducing SCI, followed by administration of MSC-EVs through various routes, most commonly intravenous (IV), at defined time points post-injury [14, 51]. Studies administered MSC-sEVs intravenously at 7 days post-SCI, employing a fractionated dosing regimen over three consecutive days to mimic the sustained release profile believed to occur from parent MSCs lodged in the lungs [14, 15].

Following intravenous infusion, a significant portion of MSC-EVs is often initially trapped in organs like the lungs, liver, and spleen, which aligns with general EV biodistribution patterns [16]. Despite this initial peripheral sequestration, crucial findings demonstrated that sEVs released by IV-delivered MSCs, or directly infused MSC-sEVs, can indeed traffic to the site of spinal cord injury [14]. This observation was further corroborated in a subsequent study utilizing human MSC-sEVs (hMSC-sEVs), where labeled hMSC-sEVs were detected at the SCI lesion site following IV administration [15].

An important aspect of this trafficking is the cellular targeting within the injury microenvironment. Both rat and human MSC-sEVs have been shown to be selectively taken up by M2-like macrophages within the injured spinal cord [14, 15]. This specific interaction with M2 macrophages is significant, as these cells play crucial roles in resolving inflammation and promoting tissue repair. The colocalization of labeled sEV hotspots with the M2 macrophage marker CD206 and the exosome marker CD63 provides strong evidence for this targeted uptake [14, 15].

The therapeutic efficacy of MSC-EVs in SCI is attributed to a confluence of intricate mechanisms that collectively foster a pro-regenerative microenvironment. A prominent mechanism is potent immunomodulation, primarily through interaction with macrophages at the injury site. MSC-EVs promote a shift in macrophage polarization from a pro-inflammatory M1 phenotype toward an anti-inflammatory and reparative M2 phenotype, evidenced by increased expression of M2 markers and decreased M1 markers at the lesion site following MSC-EV treatment [14, 15, 52, 53].

Another critical mechanism involves the repair and stabilization of the BSCB. MSC-EVs effectively restore BSCB function through multiple mechanisms. They stabilize the barrier by restoring tight junction proteins, reducing BSCB permeability, and improving endothelial-pericyte association, which contributes to better vascular stability [14, 51, 54]. Additionally, MSC-EVs downregulate harmful molecules such as endothelin-1 (ET-1) and matrix metalloproteinases (MMP-2, MMP-9), both known to participate in BSCB breakdown following spinal cord injury [54]. Furthermore, MSC-EVs regulate pericytes by suppressing their migration through the NF-κB p65 signaling pathway, which helps maintain BSCB integrity and reduces vascular leakage [51]. The therapeutic equivalence of appropriately dosed MSC-EVs to whole MSCs in SCI models, as shown regarding BSCB integrity and functional recovery, supports their development as a potent cell-free alternative [14]. The consistent evidence for improved locomotor recovery and associated mechanistic insights across multiple studies provides a strong rationale for further investigating MSC-EVs as a therapeutic modality for human SCI.

3.4 MSC-EVs and neural plasticity

While Section 2.3 established that MSCs promote neural plasticity through paracrine mechanisms, emerging evidence indicates that MSC-EVs are key mediators of these plasticity-promoting effects. MSC-EVs carry specific molecular cargo that directly induces synaptic remodeling and circuit reorganization, providing a cell-free approach to enhance neural plasticity following SCI.

Building on the enhanced corticospinal tract networks observed with MSC therapy, recent studies suggest that EVs may be primary mediators of these structural changes. MSC-EVs have been shown to accumulate specifically at sites of axonal damage, where they release cargo that promotes growth cone formation and axonal extension [55, 56]. Time-lapse imaging studies reveal that EV uptake by damaged neurons coincides with increased axonal sprouting and the formation of new synaptic connections within 48–72 hours [55].

MicroRNAs in MSC-EVs are increasingly recognized as important regulators of neural plasticity, influencing gene expression and cellular communication in the nervous system. MicroRNAs are expressed transiently and locally in neurons, responding to neuronal activity and environmental cues. This enables precise control of local protein synthesis, essential for synaptic plasticity and memory formation [57]. Among these, miR-133b enriched in MSC-EVs enhance neural plasticity and functional recovery after brain injury [58]. Additionally, miR-124-3p promotes the expression of doublecortin and β-III tubulin, facilitating cytoskeletal reorganization necessary for synaptic remodeling [59]. Furthermore, miR-26-a in MSC-EVs activates the PTEN/mTOR pathway, promoting protein synthesis required for long-term potentiation and synaptic strengthening [60].

MSC-EVs represent a concentrated delivery system for plasticity-promoting microRNAs that orchestrate neural repair at multiple levels—from cytoskeletal reorganization to synaptic protein synthesis. This targeted molecular approach provides a cell-free alternative to MSC therapy, offering precise temporal and spatial control over neural plasticity enhancement while maintaining the therapeutic benefits observed with whole-cell transplantation in SCI models.

4. Clinical applications

4.1 Current clinical trials of MSC cellular therapy

Numerous clinical trials and case series have explored MSCs for SCI, employing diverse cell sources, doses, and administration routes, including intramedullary [61–63] and intrathecal delivery (**Table 1**) [64–66].

A notable contribution is a phase 2, open-label, single-arm study involving 13 patients with subacute SCI [22]. In this trial, autologous bone marrow-derived MSCs, expanded in autologous serum under Good Manufacturing Practice (GMP) conditions, were administered intravenously. The use of autologous serum for expansion is suggested to support rapid growth and maintain a less differentiated cell phenotype [23].

The primary endpoints of this SCI study were safety and feasibility, with neurological function assessed via the American Spinal Injury Association Impairment Scale (ASIA), International Standards for Neurological and Functional Classification of Spinal Cord Injury (ISCSCI-92), and the Spinal Cord Independence Measure (SCIM-III) [22]. In this case series, 12 out of 13 patients exhibited neurological improvement in ASIA grade at 6 months post-MSC infusion, with shifts observed across different initial ASIA classifications. Notably, improvement was seen as early as 1 day post-infusion for some patients initially classified as ASIA C. Furthermore, improvements were documented in ISCSCI-92 motor and sensory scores and SCIM-III scores, which measure independence in activities of daily living, in all patients at the six-month follow-up.

Systematic reviews and meta-analyses encompassing various MSC transplantation approaches for SCI suggest potential benefits in motor and sensory recovery, although heterogeneity in study designs and outcome measures complicate definitive conclusions [67]. More recent analyses continue to highlight the overall safety of MSC transplantation but emphasize the need for larger, randomized controlled trials (RCTs) to unequivocally establish efficacy and standardize treatment protocols [68, 69]. Recent evidence also supports MSC therapy for chronic SCI, documenting significant functional improvements, including increased motor and SCIM-III scores, following MSC infusion in patients with chronic injuries [60].

The safety of MSC administration in human SCI patients has been a primary focus of numerous clinical investigations. The 13-case series reported no serious adverse events associated with the intravenous infusion of autologous, auto-serum expanded MSCs [22]. Adverse events that did occur, such as anemia following peripheral blood

Trial ID/ Reference	Phase	Design	No. of patients	Injury characteristics	MSC source	Route	Timing (post-injury)	Follow-up	Key efficacy findings
Hirota et al. [21]	— (case series)	Non-RCT, single-arm	7	Chronic (AIS C–D, 1.3–27 years)	Autologous BM-MSC	IV	Mean chronic phase	6 months	Significant functional & QOL gains; 1/7 improved AIS grade
Mendonça et al. [61]	I	Non-RCT, single-arm	14	Chronic (>6 months), complete (ASIA A), thoracic/lumbar	Autologous BM-MSC	Intralesional	>6 months	6 months	7 of 14 subjects improved to AIS B/C. 8 showed motor function recovery, and 9 showed urologic function improvement.
Dai et al. [62]	N/A	Randomized controlled trial	20 (Tx)/20 (Ctrl)	Chronic (>1 year), complete (AIS A), cervical	Autologous BM-MSC	Perilesional	>1 year	6 months	50% of Tx group showed clinical improvement; 45% improved from AIS A→B. ASIA scores significantly improved vs. Ctrl.
Oh et al. [63]	III	Non-RCT, single-arm	16	Chronic (>1 year), ASIA B, cervical	Autologous BM-MSC	Intramedullary + Subdural	>1 year	6 months	Limited efficacy. Motor improvement in 2 of 16 patients, but did not meet efficacy criteria.
Satti et al. [64]	I	Non-RCT, single-arm	9	Chronic (>6 months) & subacute (<6 months), complete (ASIA A), thoracic	Autologous BM-MSC	Intrathecal	Chronic & subacute	≥1 year	Safety confirmed. No serious adverse events. No conclusions on efficacy.
Honmou et al. [22]	II	Non-RCT, single-arm	13	Chronic (AIS A–C)	Autologous BM-MSC	IV	1.3–27 years	6 months	12/13 improved ≥ 1 AIS grade; ISCSCI-92 & SCIM-III scores ↑

Summary of clinical trials investigating Mesenchymal Stem/Stromal (MSC) therapy for patients with spinal cord injury (SCI) from 2021 to 2024. The table outlines trial design, patient characteristics, MSC source, administration route, treatment timing, follow-up period, and key efficacy outcomes. AIS: ASIA (American Spinal Injury Association) Impairment Scale, BM: bone marrow, UC: umbilical cord, AD: adipose-derived, WJ: Wharton's jelly, IV: intravenous, IT: intrathecal, QOL: quality of life, SCIM: Spinal Cord Independence Measure.

Table 1.
Clinical trials of mesenchymal stem/stromal therapy for spinal cord injury.

collection and local pain at the bone marrow aspiration site, were protocol-related and occurred before MSC infusion, indicating no MSC-related adverse events in that study cohort. Importantly, no patients developed CNS tumors, abnormal cell growth, or neurological deterioration during the follow-up period [22].

Similarly, in a study of chronic SCI patients, no serious adverse events were reported, further supporting the safety of systemic MSC administration [21]. These findings are consistent with broader systematic reviews of MSC therapies across various conditions, which generally conclude that MSC administration is well-tolerated [68, 70, 71].

4.2 Current clinical trials of MSC-EV therapy

Clinical trials investigating MSC-EVs are increasing, but the field faces challenges related to standardization, potency testing, and consistent therapeutic outcomes.

MSC-EVs are the most common cell source in EV-based clinical trials, accounting for about two-thirds of registered studies. These trials target a broad spectrum of conditions, with respiratory illnesses such as COVID-19 and acute respiratory distress syndrome being the most frequent indications. Controlled trials are increasing, with thousands of participants anticipated to receive MSC-EVs in ongoing studies [72, 73]. Beyond respiratory diseases, MSC-EVs are being explored for autoimmune and inflammatory diseases including graft-versus-host disease, multiple sclerosis, and lupus, as well as neurodegenerative disorders and various applications in tissue repair [74–76].

Despite promising results from animal studies, several challenges limit the clinical translation of MSC-EVs. There is significant variability in MSC-EV preparations, even when produced using standardized protocols. This functional heterogeneity necessitates potency testing for each batch before clinical use [73, 77, 78]. Developing robust, disease-relevant potency assays is complex due to the diverse mechanisms of action and the influence of manufacturing conditions. Regulatory-compliant assays and consistent product characterization are needed to ensure safety and efficacy [73, 77–79]. Furthermore, many trials lack detailed reporting on EV isolation and characterization methods, and few consider EV subpopulations, limiting reproducibility and translational progress [76].

Looking forward, several approaches may address these limitations and accelerate clinical translation. Combining data from ongoing trials through meta-analysis could provide sufficient power to detect clinically meaningful effects, such as mortality reduction [72]. Advances in identifying and enriching specific EV subpopulations may enable more targeted and effective therapies [76]. Addressing scalability, batch consistency, and regulatory requirements will be crucial for clinical translation and market approval of MSC-EV therapies [76, 79].

In summary, MSC-EVs represent a rapidly advancing area in clinical research, showing promise for immune modulation, tissue repair, and neuroprotection. However, challenges in standardization, potency testing, and methodological rigor must be addressed to realize their full therapeutic potential and ensure safe, effective clinical application.

5. Comparison of MSCs and MSC-EVs

MSCs and their secreted extracellular vesicles (MSC-EVs) represent two promising but fundamentally different therapeutic approaches for conditions such as spinal cord injury. While MSCs have been extensively studied for their regenerative capabilities, MSC-EVs have emerged as an alternative that may offer similar benefits with potentially fewer complications. Both originate from the same cellular source but differ significantly in their composition, mechanism of action, safety profile, and practical considerations for clinical use. Understanding these key differences is essential for researchers and clinicians to determine the most appropriate therapeutic strategy for specific applications and patient populations.

5.1 Ethical and safety challenges

The transition from cellular to vesicular therapies introduces fundamentally different ethical and safety considerations that impact clinical translation. MSC therapies face complex ethical challenges beginning with cell sourcing. Autologous MSCs require invasive bone marrow or adipose tissue harvesting and weeks of expansion, making them impractical for acute SCI treatment [22]. Allogeneic sources, particularly from perinatal tissues like umbilical cord and placenta, raise ethical questions about informed consent, commercialization of biological materials, and equitable access to donor tissues [80]. While MSC-EVs partially circumvent these issues through large-scale production from established cell lines, the use of immortalized or genetically modified cells for EV production remains largely unexplored in the literature and may introduce new ethical considerations.

Immunogenicity profiles differ significantly between the two therapies. Although MSC-EVs are generally considered less immunogenic than parent cells, emerging evidence suggests they may carry donor-specific MHC molecules. However, it remains unclear whether these molecules can elicit alloimmune responses, particularly with repeated administration [81]. Unlike MSCs, which actively suppress immune responses through dynamic cell-cell interactions, EVs lack this adaptive capability, potentially leading to antibody formation and reduced efficacy over time. Nevertheless, MSC-EVs offer a crucial safety advantage by eliminating tumorigenic risks inherent to cellular therapies. While MSCs retain theoretical risks of malignant transformation after extensive expansion, acellular EVs cannot proliferate or form ectopic tissues [82].

The regulatory landscape presents distinct challenges for each therapy type. MSCs are classified as advanced therapy medicinal products with established guidelines in both Europe and the United States. In contrast, MSC-EVs lack clear regulatory classification, as they do not fit neatly into existing categories for drugs, biologics, or cell therapies [83]. This regulatory ambiguity complicates GMP compliance, as EV heterogeneity resists standardization, and current quality metrics such as particle concentration may not predict therapeutic efficacy. Furthermore, biodistribution studies reveal that intravenously administered EVs rapidly accumulate in the liver, spleen, and lungs, with detectable presence for days to weeks after administration, though the long-term implications of this organ accumulation remain poorly understood [16, 84].

5.2 Administration routes

MSCs are typically administered through local injection directly into the affected area or via intravenous injection into blood vessels, with options potentially limited by concerns about cell viability and engraftment. MSC-EVs allow for broader administration methods due to their smaller size and acellular nature, including intravenous administration and intrathecal administration into cerebrospinal fluid, potentially enabling better access to target tissues.

5.3 Storage and transport conditions

MSCs require strict temperature control and special measures to maintain cell viability during storage and transport as they are living cells, creating logistical challenges for clinical applications and increasing costs. MSC-EVs offer significant advantages in this regard, as they can be preserved by freeze-drying methods, and their acellular nature makes storage and transport relatively easier and may extend shelf life, potentially improving clinical applicability.

5.4 Quality control parameters

For MSCs, quality control involves evaluating cell viability, proliferation capacity, and differentiation potential into specific cell types to ensure the therapeutic potential of the cells being administered. Quality control for MSC-EVs focuses on different metrics, including particle size and number, as well as characterization of the proteins and nucleic acids contained within the vesicles, which helps ensure consistent bioactivity.

5.5 Manufacturing process

The manufacturing process for MSCs involves complex steps such as cell culture, expansion, and harvesting the desired number of cells, requiring specialized facilities and expertise. The production of MSC-EVs is relatively simpler compared to handling MSCs themselves, as after MSC culture, the process involves separation and purification of EVs, which may be more amenable to standardization and scale-up for clinical applications.

Taken together, while both MSCs and MSC-EVs demonstrate therapeutic potential for SCI treatment, MSC-EVs offer distinct advantages including enhanced safety profiles, elimination of tumorigenic risks, simplified storage and transport, and broader administration routes. However, the successful clinical translation of either approach requires addressing specific challenges—MSCs face ethical concerns and safety risks associated with living cells, while MSC-EVs confront regulatory ambiguity and standardization difficulties. The choice between these therapies will ultimately depend on balancing therapeutic efficacy with practical considerations for each specific clinical application.

6. Conclusion

This comprehensive review demonstrates the significant therapeutic potential of both MSCs and MSC-EVs for spinal cord injury treatment. The evolution from cellular to vesicular approaches represents a paradigm shift in regenerative medicine, with MSC-EVs offering advantages in safety, storage, and administration while maintaining therapeutic efficacy through similar mechanisms of immunomodulation and BSCB repair. While clinical evidence supports the safety of MSC therapies, standardization challenges in MSC-EV preparation must be addressed to fully realize their therapeutic potential. The continued refinement of these approaches, particularly focusing on optimized delivery methods and potency assays, will be crucial for successful clinical translation and improved outcomes for SCI patients.

Acknowledgements

Artificial intelligence (AI) through Microsoft Copilot was utilized to correct English and grammar mistakes.

Author details

Masahito Nakazaki[1,2,3]

1 Department of Neural Regenerative Medicine, Research Institute for Frontier Medicine, Sapporo Medical University School of Medicine, Sapporo, Hokkaido, Japan

2 Department of Neurology, Yale University School of Medicine, New Haven, Connecticut, USA

3 Center for Neuroscience and Regeneration Research, VA Connecticut Healthcare System, West Haven, Connecticut, USA

*Address all correspondence to: nakazaki@sapmed.ac.jp

References

[1] Dewan MC, Rattani A, Gupta S, Baticulon RE, Hung YC, Punchak M, et al. Estimating the global incidence of traumatic brain injury. Journal of Neurosurgery. 2019;**130**(4):1080-1097

[2] Lynch J, Cahalan R. The impact of spinal cord injury on the quality of life of primary family caregivers: A literature review. Spinal Cord. 2017;**55**(11):964-978

[3] Zhou R, Li J, Chen Z, Wang R, Shen Y, Zhang R, et al. Pathological hemodynamic changes and leukocyte transmigration disrupt the blood-spinal cord barrier after spinal cord injury. Journal of Neuroinflammation. 2023;**20**(1):118

[4] Jin LY, Li J, Wang KF, Xia WW, Zhu ZQ, Wang CR, et al. Blood-spinal cord barrier in spinal cord injury: A review. Journal of Neurotrauma. 2021;**38**(9):1203-1224

[5] Figley SA, Khosravi R, Legasto JM, Tseng YF, Fehlings MG. Characterization of vascular disruption and blood-spinal cord barrier permeability following traumatic spinal cord injury. Journal of Neurotrauma. 2014;**31**(6):541-552

[6] Matsushita T, Lankford KL, Arroyo EJ, Sasaki M, Neyazi M, Radtke C, et al. Diffuse and persistent blood-spinal cord barrier disruption after contusive spinal cord injury rapidly recovers following intravenous infusion of bone marrow mesenchymal stem cells. Experimental Neurology. 2015;**267**:152-164

[7] Ahuja CS, Wilson JR, Nori S, Kotter MRN, Druschel C, Curt A, et al. Traumatic spinal cord injury. Nature Reviews. Disease Primers. 2017;**3**:17018

[8] Schwab ME, Strittmatter SM. Nogo limits neural plasticity and recovery from injury. Current Opinion in Neurobiology. 2014;**27**:53-60

[9] Bradbury EJ, Moon LD, Popat RJ, King VR, Bennett GS, Patel PN, et al. Chondroitinase ABC promotes functional recovery after spinal cord injury. Nature. 2002;**416**(6881):636-640

[10] Honmou O, Onodera R, Sasaki M, Waxman SG, Kocsis JD. Mesenchymal stem cells: Therapeutic outlook for stroke. Trends in Molecular Medicine. 2012;**18**(5):292-297

[11] Prockop DJ, Oh JY. Mesenchymal stem/stromal cells (MSCs): Role as guardians of inflammation. Molecular Therapy. 2012;**20**(1):14-20

[12] Zhou Y, Yamamoto Y, Xiao Z, Ochiya T. The immunomodulatory functions of mesenchymal stromal/stem cells mediated via paracrine activity. Journal of Clinical Medicine. 2019;**8**(7):1025-1042

[13] Alvites R, Branquinho M, Sousa AC, Lopes B, Sousa P, Mauricio AC. Mesenchymal stem/stromal cells and their paracrine activity-immunomodulation mechanisms and how to influence the therapeutic potential. Pharmaceutics. 9 Feb 2022;**14**(2):381

[14] Nakazaki M, Morita T, Lankford KL, Askenase PW, Kocsis JD. Small extracellular vesicles released by infused mesenchymal stromal cells target M2 macrophages and promote TGF-beta upregulation, microvascular stabilization and functional recovery in a rodent model of severe spinal cord injury. Journal of Extracellular Vesicles. 2021;**10**(11):e12137

[15] Nakazaki M, Lankford KL, Yamamoto H, Mae Y, Kocsis JD. Human

mesenchymal stem-derived extracellular vesicles improve body growth and motor function following severe spinal cord injury in rat. Clinical and Translational Medicine. 2023;**13**(6):e1284

[16] Lankford KL, Arroyo EJ, Nazimek K, Bryniarski K, Askenase PW, Kocsis JD. Intravenously delivered mesenchymal stem cell-derived exosomes target M2-type macrophages in the injured spinal cord. PLoS One. 2018;**13**(1):e0190358

[17] Kuang Y, Zheng X, Zhang L, Ai X, Venkataramani V, Kilic E, et al. Adipose-derived mesenchymal stem cells reduce autophagy in stroke mice by extracellular vesicle transfer of miR-25. Journal of Extracellular Vesicles. 2020;**10**(1):e12024

[18] Dominici M, Le Blanc K, Mueller I, Slaper-Cortenbach I, Marini F, Krause D, et al. Minimal criteria for defining multipotent mesenchymal stromal cells. The International Society for Cellular Therapy position statement. Cytotherapy. 2006;**8**(4):315-317

[19] Pittenger MF, Mackay AM, Beck SC, Jaiswal RK, Douglas R, Mosca JD, et al. Multilineage potential of adult human mesenchymal stem cells. Science. 1999;**284**(5411):143-147

[20] Meirelles Lda S, Fontes AM, Covas DT, Caplan AI. Mechanisms involved in the therapeutic properties of mesenchymal stem cells. Cytokine & Growth Factor Reviews. 2009;**20**(5-6):419-427

[21] Hirota R, Sasaki M, Iyama S, Kurihara K, Fukushi R, Obara H, et al. Intravenous infusion of autologous mesenchymal stem cells expanded in auto serum for chronic spinal cord injury patients: A case series. Journal of Clinical Medicine. 11 Oct 2024;**13**(20):6072

[22] Honmou O, Yamashita T, Morita T, Oshigiri T, Hirota R, Iyama S, et al. Intravenous infusion of auto serum-expanded autologous mesenchymal stem cells in spinal cord injury patients: 13 case series. Clinical Neurology and Neurosurgery. 2021;**203**:106565

[23] Honmou O, Houkin K, Matsunaga T, Niitsu Y, Ishiai S, Onodera R, et al. Intravenous administration of auto serum-expanded autologous mesenchymal stem cells in stroke. Brain. 2011;**134**(Pt. 6):1790-1807

[24] Fontaine MJ, Shih H, Schafer R, Pittenger MF. Unraveling the mesenchymal stromal cells' paracrine immunomodulatory effects. Transfusion Medicine Reviews. 2016;**30**(1):37-43

[25] Nakazaki M, Sasaki M, Kataoka-Sasaki Y, Oka S, Suzuki J, Sasaki Y, et al. Intravenous infusion of mesenchymal stem cells improves impaired cognitive function in a cerebral small vessel disease model. Neuroscience. 2019;**408**:361-377

[26] Maccario R, Podesta M, Moretta A, Cometa A, Comoli P, Montagna D, et al. Interaction of human mesenchymal stem cells with cells involved in alloantigen-specific immune response favors the differentiation of CD4+ T-cell subsets expressing a regulatory/suppressive phenotype. Haematologica. 2005;**90**(4):516-525

[27] Sze SK, de Kleijn DP, Lai RC, Khia Way Tan E, Zhao H, Yeo KS, et al. Elucidating the secretion proteome of human embryonic stem cell-derived mesenchymal stem cells. Molecular & Cellular Proteomics. 2007;**6**(10):1680-1689

[28] Gangadaran P, Rajendran RL, Lee HW, Kalimuthu S, Hong CM, Jeong SY, et al. Extracellular vesicles from

mesenchymal stem cells activates VEGF receptors and accelerates recovery of hindlimb ischemia. Journal of Controlled Release. 2017;**264**:112-126

[29] Sasaki M, Radtke C, Tan AM, Zhao P, Hamada H, Houkin K, et al. BDNF-hypersecreting human mesenchymal stem cells promote functional recovery, axonal sprouting, and protection of corticospinal neurons after spinal cord injury. The Journal of Neuroscience. 2009;**29**(47):14932-14941

[30] Zheng W, Honmou O, Miyata K, Harada K, Suzuki J, Liu H, et al. Therapeutic benefits of human mesenchymal stem cells derived from bone marrow after global cerebral ischemia. Brain Research. 2010;**1310**:8-16

[31] Nandoe Tewarie RD, Yu J, Seidel J, Rahiem ST, Hurtado A, Tsui BM, et al. Positron emission tomography for serial imaging of the contused adult rat spinal cord. Molecular Imaging. 2010;**9**(2):108-116

[32] Basso DM, Beattie MS, Bresnahan JC. Graded histological and locomotor outcomes after spinal cord contusion using the NYU weight-drop device versus transection. Experimental Neurology. 1996;**139**(2):244-256

[33] Osaka M, Honmou O, Murakami T, Nonaka T, Houkin K, Hamada H, et al. Intravenous administration of mesenchymal stem cells derived from bone marrow after contusive spinal cord injury improves functional outcome. Brain Research. 2010;**1343**:226-235

[34] Nakajima H, Uchida K, Guerrero AR, Watanabe S, Sugita D, Takeura N, et al. Transplantation of mesenchymal stem cells promotes an alternative pathway of macrophage activation and functional recovery after spinal cord injury. Journal of Neurotrauma. 2012;**29**(8):1614-1625

[35] Kim JW, Ha KY, Molon JN, Kim YH. Bone marrow-derived mesenchymal stem cell transplantation for chronic spinal cord injury in rats: Comparative study between intralesional and intravenous transplantation. Spine (Phila Pa 1976). 2013;**38**(17):E1065-E1074

[36] Morita T, Sasaki M, Kataoka-Sasaki Y, Nakazaki M, Nagahama H, Oka S, et al. Intravenous infusion of mesenchymal stem cells promotes functional recovery in a model of chronic spinal cord injury. Neuroscience. 2016;**335**:221-231

[37] Oshigiri T, Sasaki T, Sasaki M, Kataoka-Sasaki Y, Nakazaki M, Oka S, et al. Intravenous infusion of mesenchymal stem cells alters motor cortex gene expression in a rat model of acute spinal cord injury. Journal of Neurotrauma. 2019;**36**(3):411-420

[38] Hirota R, Sasaki M, Kataoka-Sasaki Y, Oshigiri T, Kurihara K, Fukushi R, et al. Enhanced network in corticospinal tracts after infused mesenchymal stem cells in spinal cord injury. Journal of Neurotrauma. 2022;**39**(23-24):1665-1677

[39] Park HJ, Oh SH, Kim HN, Jung YJ, Lee PH. Mesenchymal stem cells enhance alpha-synuclein clearance via M2 microglia polarization in experimental and human parkinsonian disorder. Acta Neuropathologica. 2016;**132**(5):685-701

[40] Sasaki Y, Sasaki M, Kataoka-Sasaki Y, Nakazaki M, Nagahama H, Suzuki J, et al. Synergic effects of rehabilitation and intravenous infusion of mesenchymal stem cells after stroke in rats. Physical Therapy. 2016;**96**(11):1791-1798

[41] De Feo D, Merlini A, Laterza C, Martino G. Neural stem cell transplantation in central nervous system

disorders: From cell replacement to neuroprotection. Current Opinion in Neurology. 2012;**25**(3):322-333

[42] Cao Q, Zhang YP, Iannotti C, DeVries WH, Xu XM, Shields CB, et al. Functional and electrophysiological changes after graded traumatic spinal cord injury in adult rat. Experimental Neurology. 2005;**191**(Suppl. 1):S3-S16

[43] Neuhuber B, Timothy Himes B, Shumsky JS, Gallo G, Fischer I. Axon growth and recovery of function supported by human bone marrow stromal cells in the injured spinal cord exhibit donor variations. Brain Research. 2005;**1035**(1):73-85

[44] Lee RH, Pulin AA, Seo MJ, Kota DJ, Ylostalo J, Larson BL, et al. Intravenous hMSCs improve myocardial infarction in mice because cells embolized in lung are activated to secrete the anti-inflammatory protein TSG-6. Cell Stem Cell. 2009;**5**(1):54-63

[45] Huang JH, Yin XM, Xu Y, Xu CC, Lin X, Ye FB, et al. Systemic Administration of Exosomes Released from mesenchymal stromal cells attenuates apoptosis, inflammation, and promotes angiogenesis after spinal cord injury in rats. Journal of Neurotrauma. 2017;**34**(24):3388-3396

[46] Song Y, Dou H, Li X, Zhao X, Li Y, Liu D, et al. Exosomal miR-146a contributes to the enhanced therapeutic efficacy of interleukin-1beta-primed mesenchymal stem cells against sepsis. Stem Cells. 2017;**35**(5):1208-1221

[47] Welsh JA, Goberdhan DCI, O'Driscoll L, Buzas EI, Blenkiron C, Bussolati B, et al. Minimal information for studies of extracellular vesicles (MISEV2023): From basic to advanced approaches. Journal of Extracellular Vesicles. 2024;**13**(2):e12404

[48] Volarevic V, Markovic BS, Gazdic M, Volarevic A, Jovicic N, Arsenijevic N, et al. Ethical and safety issues of stem cell-based therapy. International Journal of Medical Sciences. 2018;**15**(1):36-45

[49] Sokolova V, Ludwig AK, Hornung S, Rotan O, Horn PA, Epple M, et al. Characterisation of exosomes derived from human cells by nanoparticle tracking analysis and scanning electron microscopy. Colloids and Surfaces. B, Biointerfaces. 2011;**87**(1):146-150

[50] Witwer KW, Van Balkom BWM, Bruno S, Choo A, Dominici M, Gimona M, et al. Defining mesenchymal stromal cell (MSC)-derived small extracellular vesicles for therapeutic applications. Journal of Extracellular Vesicles. 2019;**8**(1):1609206

[51] Lu Y, Zhou Y, Zhang R, Wen L, Wu K, Li Y, et al. Bone mesenchymal stem cell-derived extracellular vesicles promote recovery following spinal cord injury via improvement of the integrity of the blood-spinal cord barrier. Frontiers in Neuroscience. 2019;**13**:209

[52] Li M, Zhang T, Li P, Luan Z, Liu J, Wang Y, et al. IL-4-primed human umbilical cord mesenchymal stem cells-derived extracellular vesicles facilitate recovery in spinal cord injury via the miR-21-5p/PDCD4-mediated shifting of macrophage M1/M2 polarization. Life Sciences. 2025;**364**:123441

[53] Liu W, Tang P, Wang J, Ye W, Ge X, Rong Y, et al. Extracellular vesicles derived from melatonin-preconditioned mesenchymal stem cells containing USP29 repair traumatic spinal cord injury by stabilizing NRF2. Journal of Pineal Research. 2021;**71**(4):e12769

[54] Xue C, Ma X, Guan X, Feng H, Zheng M, Yang X. Small extracellular vesicles derived from umbilical cord

mesenchymal stem cells repair blood-spinal cord barrier disruption after spinal cord injury through down-regulation of Endothelin-1 in rats. PeerJ. 2023;**11**:e16311

[55] Zhang Y, Chopp M, Liu XS, Katakowski M, Wang X, Tian X, et al. Exosomes derived from mesenchymal stromal cells promote axonal growth of cortical neurons. Molecular Neurobiology. 2017;**54**(4):2659-2673

[56] Martins LF, Costa RO, Pedro JR, Aguiar P, Serra SC, Teixeira FG, et al. Mesenchymal stem cells secretome-induced axonal outgrowth is mediated by BDNF. Scientific Reports. 2017;**7**(1):4153

[57] Vo NK, Cambronne XA, Goodman RH. MicroRNA pathways in neural development and plasticity. Current Opinion in Neurobiology. 2010;**20**(4):457-465

[58] Xin H, Wang F, Li Y, Lu QE, Cheung WL, Zhang Y, et al. Secondary release of exosomes from astrocytes contributes to the increase in neural plasticity and improvement of functional recovery after stroke in rats treated with exosomes harvested from MicroRNA 133b-overexpressing multipotent mesenchymal stromal cells. Cell Transplantation. 2017;**26**(2):243-257

[59] Doeppner TR, Herz J, Gorgens A, Schlechter J, Ludwig AK, Radtke S, et al. Extracellular vesicles improve post-stroke Neuroregeneration and prevent Postischemic immunosuppression. Stem Cells Translational Medicine. 2015;**4**(10):1131-1143

[60] Chen Y, Tian Z, He L, Liu C, Wang N, Rong L, et al. Exosomes derived from miR-26a-modified MSCs promote axonal regeneration via the PTEN/AKT/mTOR pathway following spinal cord injury. Stem Cell Research & Therapy. 2021;**12**(1):224

[61] Mendonca MV, Larocca TF, de Freitas Souza BS, Villarreal CF, Silva LF, Matos AC, et al. Safety and neurological assessments after autologous transplantation of bone marrow mesenchymal stem cells in subjects with chronic spinal cord injury. Stem Cell Research & Therapy. 2014;**5**(6):126

[62] Dai G, Liu X, Zhang Z, Yang Z, Dai Y, Xu R. Transplantation of autologous bone marrow mesenchymal stem cells in the treatment of complete and chronic cervical spinal cord injury. Brain Research. 2013;**1533**:73-79

[63] Oh SK, Choi KH, Yoo JY, Kim DY, Kim SJ, Jeon SR. A phase III clinical trial showing limited efficacy of autologous mesenchymal stem cell therapy for spinal cord injury. Neurosurgery. 2016;**78**(3):436-447; discussion 47

[64] Satti HS, Waheed A, Ahmed P, Ahmed K, Akram Z, Aziz T, et al. Autologous mesenchymal stromal cell transplantation for spinal cord injury: A phase I pilot study. Cytotherapy. 2016;**18**(4):518-522

[65] Karamouzian S, Nematollahi-Mahani SN, Nakhaee N, Eskandary H. Clinical safety and primary efficacy of bone marrow mesenchymal cell transplantation in subacute spinal cord injured patients. Clinical Neurology and Neurosurgery. 2012;**114**(7):935-939

[66] Vaquero J, Zurita M, Rico MA, Bonilla C, Aguayo C, Fernandez C, et al. Repeated subarachnoid administrations of autologous mesenchymal stromal cells supported in autologous plasma improve quality of life in patients suffering incomplete spinal cord injury. Cytotherapy. 2017;**19**(3):349-359

[67] Xu P, Yang X. The efficacy and safety of mesenchymal stem cell transplantation for spinal cord injury patients: A meta-analysis and systematic review. Cell Transplantation. 2019;**28**(1):36-46

[68] Chen WC, Liu WF, Bai YY, Zhou YY, Zhang Y, Wang CM, et al. Transplantation of mesenchymal stem cells for spinal cord injury: A systematic review and network meta-analysis. Journal of Translational Medicine. 2021;**19**(1):178

[69] Muthu S, Jeyaraman M, Gulati A, Arora A. Current evidence on mesenchymal stem cell therapy for traumatic spinal cord injury: Systematic review and meta-analysis. Cytotherapy. 2021;**23**(3):186-197

[70] Lalu MM, McIntyre L, Pugliese C, Fergusson D, Winston BW, Marshall JC, et al. Safety of cell therapy with mesenchymal stromal cells (SafeCell): A systematic review and meta-analysis of clinical trials. PLoS One. 2012;**7**(10):e47559

[71] Thompson M, Mei SHJ, Wolfe D, Champagne J, Fergusson D, Stewart DJ, et al. Cell therapy with intravascular administration of mesenchymal stromal cells continues to appear safe: An updated systematic review and meta-analysis. EClinicalMedicine. 2020;**19**:100249

[72] Duong A, Parmar G, Kirkham AM, Burger D, Allan DS. Registered clinical trials investigating treatment with cell-derived extracellular vesicles: A scoping review. Cytotherapy. 2023;**25**(9):939-945

[73] Gimona M, Brizzi MF, Choo ABH, Dominici M, Davidson SM, Grillari J, et al. Critical considerations for the development of potency tests for therapeutic applications of mesenchymal stromal cell-derived small extracellular vesicles. Cytotherapy. 2021;**23**(5):373-380

[74] Lai P, Weng J, Guo L, Chen X, Du X. Novel insights into MSC-EVs therapy for immune diseases. Biomarker Research. 2019;**7**:6

[75] Varderidou-Minasian S, Lorenowicz MJ. Mesenchymal stromal/stem cell-derived extracellular vesicles in tissue repair: Challenges and opportunities. Theranostics. 2020;**10**(13):5979-5997

[76] Mizenko RR, Feaver M, Bozkurt BT, Lowe N, Nguyen B, Huang KW, et al. A critical systematic review of extracellular vesicle clinical trials. Journal of Extracellular Vesicles. 2024;**13**(10):e12510

[77] Madel RJ, Borger V, Dittrich R, Bremer M, Tertel T, Phuong NNT, et al. Independent human mesenchymal stromal cell-derived extracellular vesicle preparations differentially attenuate symptoms in an advanced murine graft-versus-host disease model. Cytotherapy. 2023;**25**(8):821-836

[78] Liu X, Wei Q, Lu L, Cui S, Ma K, Zhang W, et al. Immunomodulatory potential of mesenchymal stem cell-derived extracellular vesicles: Targeting immune cells. Frontiers in Immunology. 2023;**14**:1094685

[79] Giovannelli L, Bari E, Jommi C, Tartara F, Armocida D, Garbossa D, et al. Mesenchymal stem cell secretome and extracellular vesicles for neurodegenerative diseases: Risk-benefit profile and next steps for the market access. Bioactive Materials. 2023;**29**:16-35

[80] Zhu D, Barabadi M, McDonald C, Kusuma G, Inocencio IM, Lim R. Implications of maternal-fetal health on perinatal stem cell banking. Gene Therapy. 2024;**31**(3-4):65-73

[81] Lohan P, Treacy O, Griffin MD, Ritter T, Ryan AE. Anti-donor immune

responses elicited by allogeneic mesenchymal stem cells and their extracellular vesicles: Are we still learning? Frontiers in Immunology. 2017;**8**:1626

[82] Yeo RW, Lai RC, Zhang B, Tan SS, Yin Y, Teh BJ, et al. Mesenchymal stem cell: An efficient mass producer of exosomes for drug delivery. Advanced Drug Delivery Reviews. 2013;**65**(3):336-341

[83] Iglesias-Lopez C, Agusti A, Obach M, Vallano A. Regulatory framework for advanced therapy medicinal products in Europe and United States. Frontiers in Pharmacology. 2019;**10**:921

[84] Kang M, Jordan V, Blenkiron C, Chamley LW. Biodistribution of extracellular vesicles following administration into animals: A systematic review. Journal of Extracellular Vesicles. 2021;**10**(8):e12085

Chapter 2

Regenerative Therapy for Ischemic Brain Injury Using Neural Stem Cells: Mechanisms, Enhancement, and Impact on Neurogenesis

Xiao Liu

Abstract

Stem cell-based therapies, particularly those involving neural stem cells (NSCs), offer great promise for the treatment of cerebral ischemia, a condition that includes ischemic stroke, cardiac arrest-induced global ischemia, and hypoxic-ischemic encephalopathy. Preclinical models demonstrate that NSC therapy can promote neuroregeneration, reduce inflammation, and improve functional recovery. However, translation into clinical application remains hindered by poor graft survival, limited integration, and adverse microenvironments. To overcome these barriers, multiple stem cell modification techniques have been developed, including metabolic glyco-engineering, genetic modification, preconditioning, and biomaterial encapsulation. This chapter reviews the pathophysiology of cerebral ischemia, the mechanisms of NSC therapy, and advanced bioengineering strategies to enhance stem cell therapeutic efficacy across different ischemic models.

Keywords: neural stem cells, ischemic stroke, cardiac arrest, hypoxic-ischemic encephalopathy, metabolic glycoengineering, genetic modification, biomaterials

1. Introduction

Ischemic brain injury is one of the most devastating neurological insults, contributing significantly to long-term morbidity and mortality worldwide. Cerebral ischemia refers to a pathological condition characterized by insufficient blood flow to the brain. This results in widespread neuronal dysfunction, impaired axonal regeneration, and irreversible cell death [1]. The three major clinical scenarios where cerebral ischemia manifests include focal ischemic stroke, global ischemia following cardiac arrest (CA), and neonatal hypoxic-ischemic encephalopathy (HIE). Each condition involves distinct anatomical and pathophysiological profiles but shares common mechanisms such as glutamate excitotoxicity, oxidative stress, inflammation [1], and breakdown of the blood-brain barrier (BBB) [2].

Despite advancements in reperfusion therapies such as thrombolysis and mechanical thrombectomy for stroke, and targeted temperature management for post-CA care, functional recovery remains limited [3]. Survivors post-CA frequently suffer from persistent cognitive deficits, memory loss, and decreased quality of life due to extensive neuronal damage [4, 5]. These injuries are particularly pronounced in the hippocampus and cerebral cortex—regions especially vulnerable to ischemia [6]. In neonatal HIE, hypothermia is the standard of care, but many infants still suffer from long-term neurological deficits [7]. Thus, there is an urgent need for regenerative strategies that can repair injured tissue and restore lost neural functions.

In this context, regenerative medicine, and particularly stem cell-based therapies, have emerged as a compelling frontier. Neural stem cells (NSCs) possess inherent neurogenic potential, offering prospects for cell differentiation, neuroprotection, and modulation of the injury microenvironment. NSCs can differentiate into neurons, astrocytes, and oligodendrocytes [8] and secrete a broad range of trophic factors that support synaptogenesis, angiogenesis, and endogenous repair processes [9]. Preclinical studies have shown that transplanted NSCs can home to sites of injury, promoted neuronal survival, and restored functional deficits [10]. However, despite these promising results, clinical translation has been slow and fraught with limitations.

Key challenges in NSC-based therapies include poor cell survival after transplantation, limited engraftment, insufficient migration toward lesion sites, and inadequate integration into host neural circuits [11]. These shortcomings are largely due to the inhospitable post-ischemic brain environment—characterized by inflammation, loss of structural extracellular matrix (ECM) support, disrupted trophic signaling, and high levels of reactive oxygen species. In addition, transplanted cells often fail to establish stable interactions with the surrounding tissue, leading to rapid clearance or apoptosis.

To overcome these limitations, various stem cell enhancement strategies have been developed. These include metabolic glycoengineering (MGE) to modify glycans on the cell surface, genetic modification to overexpress neuroprotective factors, encapsulation in biomaterials to enhance retention and integration, and preconditioning approaches to improve cell resilience. Additionally, stem cell-derived extracellular vesicles are gaining attention for their cell-free therapeutic potential.

This chapter provides a comprehensive overview of the pathophysiology of cerebral ischemia, current experimental models, the mechanisms of NSC-based neuroprotection, and delivery strategies. It focuses on how NSC-based therapies repair ischemic brain injury by promoting endogenous neurogenesis and modulating the neurogenic microenvironment. It highlights advanced cell engineering techniques to optimize stem cell therapy for different ischemic conditions and offers insights into translational challenges and future directions.

2. Pathophysiology of cerebral ischemia

Cerebral ischemia initiates a multifaceted cascade of biochemical and cellular events that differ in spatial and temporal dynamics depending on the etiology—stroke, CA-induced ischemic brain injury, or neonatal HIE. The ischemic process begins with a sudden reduction or cessation of cerebral blood flow, leading to energy failure, ionic imbalance, and excitotoxicity. Loss of ATP impairs $Na+/K+$ ATPase function, causing neuronal depolarization, intracellular calcium accumulation, and the release of excitatory neurotransmitters such as glutamate [12]. This results in excitotoxic neuronal death, particularly in vulnerable regions such as the hippocampus and cortex [13].

In the subacute phase, mitochondrial dysfunction and oxidative stress lead to the generation of reactive oxygen species and the activation of apoptotic pathways [14]. The ischemic insult also compromises the BBB [2], enabling the infiltration of peripheral immune cells and contributing to the activation of resident glial cells. Microglia become reactive and adopt pro-inflammatory phenotypes, releasing cytokines such as TNF-α, IL-1β, and IL-6, which exacerbate neuronal injury [15]. Astrocytes undergo hypertrophy and form glial scars that can hinder axonal regeneration [16].

Despite these injurious processes, the brain retains a limited capacity for repair, evidenced by increased neurogenesis in the subventricular zone (SVZ), angiogenesis in peri-infarct regions, and synaptic reorganization. However, these endogenous responses are often inadequate for meaningful recovery, necessitating exogenous intervention such as NSC transplantation.

3. Experimental models of cerebral ischemia

Experimental models have been developed to mimic different forms of ischemic brain injury and provide a critical platform to evaluate NSC therapy. These models are designed to replicate the complex pathophysiological processes that occur in human conditions, enabling researchers to study neuronal loss, glial responses, neuroinflammation, and endogenous repair mechanisms under controlled experimental settings. Among the most widely used are models of focal ischemic stroke, which reproduce occlusion of cerebral arteries leading to localized infarction; global cerebral ischemia following CA, which produces widespread brain damage due to transient whole-brain hypoperfusion; and neonatal HIE, which reflects the vulnerability of the immature brain to combined hypoxia and ischemia. Together, these preclinical systems not only provide mechanistic insights into injury progression and repair but also serve as indispensable platforms for testing the efficacy, delivery methods, and safety of emerging NSC-based interventions.

3.1 Ischemic stroke

3.1.1 Middle cerebral artery occlusion (MCAO)

This widely used rodent model mimics focal ischemic stroke by mechanically occluding the middle cerebral artery, typically using an intraluminal filament introduced through the carotid artery [17]. Occlusion can be transient, allowing reperfusion after a defined period, or permanent if the filament is left in place. This approach produces infarction in both cortical and subcortical regions, closely resembling human ischemic stroke, and is commonly employed to study ischemia-reperfusion injury, neuroprotection, and functional recovery.

3.1.2 Photothrombotic cortical stroke

This model induces focal cortical ischemia by injecting the photosensitive dye Rose Bengal followed by targeted illumination of the skull with a green light source [18]. The combination generates localized microvascular thrombosis, leading to a sharply demarcated infarct in the illuminated cortical region. It is highly reproducible and allows precise spatial control of lesion location, making it useful for studies of cortical stroke, functional recovery, and rehabilitation interventions.

3.1.3 Endothelin-1 (ET-1) vasoconstriction

This model induces focal cerebral ischemia by stereotaxically injecting the potent vasoconstrictor endothelin-1 near targeted cerebral arteries or brain regions. ET-1 causes transient vessel constriction and reduction of local blood flow, leading to ischemic injury with gradual and spontaneous reperfusion [19]. The lesion size and location can be precisely controlled by the injection site and dose, making this method versatile for modeling both cortical and subcortical strokes and for studying region-specific ischemic mechanisms and recovery.

3.2 CA-induced global cerebral ischemia

3.2.1 Asphyxial CA

This model induces global cerebral ischemia by stopping ventilation in anesthetized and intubated rodents, leading to progressive hypoxemia, hypercapnia, and eventual cardiac arrest. After a defined no-flow period, cardiopulmonary resuscitation (CPR) is performed with chest compressions, mechanical ventilation, and pharmacological support to achieve return of spontaneous circulation (ROSC) [10, 11, 20–22]. Asphyxial CA closely mimics respiratory or drowning-related CA in humans and reliably produces hippocampal and cortical neuronal injury, making it suitable for studying mechanisms of post-ischemic brain damage and neuroprotective interventions.

3.2.2 Ventricular fibrillation CA

In this model, ventricular fibrillation is electrically induced using a pacing electrode placed in the heart, leading to sudden cessation of effective circulation. After a defined period of untreated arrest, CPR with chest compressions, ventilation, defibrillation, and pharmacological support is applied to restore spontaneous circulation [23]. Ventricular fibrillation CA closely replicates the pathophysiology of sudden CA in humans due to arrhythmias and produces reproducible global cerebral ischemia, making it highly relevant for translational studies of neuroprotection and resuscitation strategies.

3.2.3 Potassium chloride (KCl)-Induced CA

This model produces rapid and reproducible CA by intravenous or intracardiac injection of KCl, which causes immediate asystole. After a predetermined ischemic interval, resuscitation is initiated with chest compressions, ventilation, and pharmacological support to restore circulation [24]. KCl-induced arrest offers precise control over arrest duration and consistently produces diffuse ischemic brain injury, particularly in vulnerable regions such as the hippocampus, though it is less physiologically representative of spontaneous human cardiac arrest.

3.3 Neonatal HIE

3.3.1 Rice-Vannucci model

This widely used neonatal HIE model is performed in postnatal day 7 rodent pups by permanent ligation of one common carotid artery followed by exposure to a hypoxic environment, typically 8% oxygen for 30–120 minutes [25]. The combined reduction in cerebral blood flow and oxygen supply produces unilateral brain injury involving the cortex, hippocampus, and striatum. It closely mimics the pathophysiology of human neonatal HIE and is considered the gold-standard model for studying mechanisms of injury and testing neuroprotective therapies.

3.3.2 Bilateral carotid artery occlusion + hypoxia

In this approach, both common carotid arteries are occluded in neonatal or juvenile rodents and combined with systemic hypoxia exposure [26]. This produces widespread, symmetric ischemic damage in hippocampal and white matter regions, modeling severe forms of HIE. It is especially useful for investigating global hypoxic-ischemic injury, though associated with higher mortality.

3.3.3 Hypoxia alone

This model involves placing neonatal rodents in a hypoxic chamber (5–8% O_2) for a prolonged period without arterial occlusion [27]. It results in diffuse, milder brain injury without a strong ischemic component. This method is simple and reproducible, making it suitable for studies of systemic hypoxia and milder neonatal encephalopathy.

3.3.4 Ischemia alone

Here, ischemic injury is induced by occlusion of cerebral or carotid arteries without hypoxia exposure [28]. This produces focal infarcts, typically in cortical and striatal regions, allowing researchers to study ischemia-specific mechanisms. It is often used as a control or complementary model to distinguish ischemic from hypoxic contributions to brain injury.

Overall, each of these models captures distinct pathophysiological features and allows for the examination of therapeutic efficacy across developmental stages and injury types. Stroke models are particularly well suited for studying focal ischemic deficits, cortical reorganization, and region-specific plasticity, offering insight into mechanisms of localized repair. CA models diffuse global ischemia, allowing investigation of diffuse injury and long-range network dysfunction. Neonatal HIE models uniquely address the immature brain, where neurodevelopmental processes interact with ischemic injury, allowing assessment of therapies in the context of growth, synaptogenesis, and white matter maturation. HIE models help evaluate interventions in the developing brain. By leveraging the complementary strengths of these platforms, researchers can systematically evaluate NSC survival, integration, and functional recovery across clinically relevant scenarios. Collectively, these models serve as indispensable bridges between basic mechanistic discoveries and clinical translation, ultimately advancing the optimization of NSC-based therapies for diverse forms of ischemic brain injury.

4. NSC therapy in ischemic brain injury

Building upon the detailed understanding of cerebral ischemia pathology and experimental models outlined above, we now explore the application of NSC therapy across different models and its repair mechanisms. NSC therapy has emerged as a promising regenerative strategy for treating ischemic brain injury due to the intrinsic properties of NSCs. These include the capacity for self-renewal, multipotent differentiation, and homing to injury sites [29]. NSCs can differentiate into the three primary neural lineages—neurons, astrocytes, and oligodendrocytes [8]—making them ideal candidates for replacing lost or damaged cells in the central nervous system.

Beyond direct cell differentiation, NSCs exert potent paracrine effects that modulate the post-ischemic environment. They secrete a variety of trophic and anti-inflammatory factors including brain-derived neurotrophic factor (BDNF), vascular endothelial growth factor (VEGF), glial-derived neurotrophic factor (GDNF), and insulin-like growth factor-1 (IGF-1) [30, 31]. These secreted factors promote angiogenesis, neurogenesis, and synaptic plasticity [9] and protect against oxidative stress [32]. Importantly, NSCs can also interface with host immune cells to dampen detrimental inflammation [22].

One of the critical features of NSCs is their ability to migrate toward injured brain regions in response to chemotactic cues [10]. Factors such as stromal-derived factor 1α (SDF-1α) [33], monocyte chemoattractant protein-1 (MCP-1) [34], and hepatocyte growth factor (HGF) [35] help guide NSCs to the site of damage. Upon arrival, NSCs can integrate into the local environment, forming connections with host neurons and contributing to the restoration of neural circuits [36].

In preclinical models of ischemic stroke, administration of NSCs have been shown to reduce infarct volume, increase endogenous neurogenesis [37], promote angiogenesis [38], enhance neural reorganization [39], and modulate neuroinflammation [40], which ultimately led to improved neurological recovery. In CA-induced global cerebral ischemia models, intracerebroventricular administration of NSCs 3 hours after ROSC improved both functional and electrophysiologic recovery, partly through modulation of the Wnt/β-catenin inflammatory pathway [10, 41]. The grafted cells also showed proliferation and migration from the SVZ compared with controls [10, 41]. Moreover, intranasal delivery of NSCs at the same time point provided great neuroprotection by regulating the TLR4/NLRP3 inflammatory pathway in vitro and in vivo [22]. Similarly, in neonatal HIE models, transplantation of NSCs has been shown to preserve oligodendrocyte survival and promote remyelination, thereby improving cognitive and motor outcomes [42, 43].

Despite encouraging results, several limitations remain. The ischemic environment is often inhospitable to graft survival, with high levels of oxidative stress, inflammation, and poor ECM support [11]. Engrafted NSCs may exhibit limited survival and differentiation unless modified to enhance resilience and trophic factor secretion. Furthermore, efficient delivery remains a challenge, especially in acute settings where timing is critical and invasive procedures may be contraindicated.

To overcome these barriers, several enhancement strategies have been developed (see **Table 1**). These include MGE, which modifies the glycocalyx to improve cell adhesion, migration, and interaction with the ECM [44, 45]. Genetic modification allows overexpression of anti-apoptotic or pro-neurogenic genes [46]. Preconditioning with hypoxia or inflammatory stimuli can enhance NSC resistance to hostile environments [51]. Encapsulation in biocompatible hydrogels improves graft localization and survival, while simultaneously delivering growth factors in a controlled manner [47, 48]. Recent studies also highlight the potential of NSC-derived extracellular vesicles, including exosomes and microvesicles, which carry proteins, lipids, and RNAs that mediate neuroprotection [50]. Extracellular vesicles are cell-free and have lower safety concerns, making them attractive for clinical applications.

Strategy	Advantages	Disadvantages	Potential impact on neurogenesis/Brain development
Metabolic glycoengineering [44, 45]	Simple, non-genetic, broad effects on adhesion, survival, and differentiation, modulates signaling pathways	Requires optimization for specific cell types, potential for off-target glycosylation, good manufacturing practice-grade precursor availability	Enhances NSC adhesion and integration into neural niches; activates Wnt/β-catenin signaling promoting neurogenesis
Genetic Modification [46]	Precise targeting of specific genes, potential for long-term effects	Ethical concerns, potential for insertional mutagenesis, immunogenicity, regulatory hurdles, complex and high cost	Overexpression of BDNF, GDNF, or IL-10 supports neuronal survival, differentiation, and synaptic maturation
Biomaterial Encapsulation [47, 48]	Enhanced survival and localized delivery, protection from immune response	Limited control over differentiation, potential for foreign body reaction, scalability challenges, difficult to assess the performance	Provides structural cues supporting neuroblast migration, axonal growth, and network formation
Preconditioning with Factors [49]	Relatively simple, can enhance specific functions (e.g., neurotrophic factor secretion	Transient effects, requires careful optimization of factor combinations and dosages, inconsistent results and off target effect	Upregulates survival and angiogenic pathways; primes NSCs for enhanced neuronal differentiation post-engraftment
Extracellular Vesicles [50]	Cell-free approach, reduced risk of tumorigenicity, carry bioactive molecules (proteins, RNAs, and lipids)	Limited yield and standardization, challenges in large-scale isolation and purification, short half-life in vivo, incomplete understanding of mechanisms	Transfer neurotrophic and developmental factors that enhance endogenous neurogenesis and synaptic remodeling

Table 1.
Comparison of stem cell therapy enhancement strategies.

Overall, NSC therapy represents a versatile platform for addressing the multifactorial damage caused by cerebral ischemia. Continued efforts in bioengineering and delivery optimization are essential to fully realize its therapeutic potential and ensure translation from bench to bedside.

5. Delivery strategies for NSC therapy

The therapeutic efficacy of NSC transplantation is significantly influenced by the route of administration. Effective delivery strategies must optimize cell survival, migration, integration, and distribution within the target regions, while minimizing invasiveness and potential complications. Several delivery methods have been evaluated in preclinical models, including intracerebroventricular, intranasal, intracranial, intravenous, and intra-arterial routes [29]. Each approach has its own advantages and limitations.

5.1 Intracerebroventricular delivery

This method involves direct injection of NSCs into the cerebral ventricles, allowing cells to diffuse along the cerebrospinal fluid and migrate toward injury sites. Intracerebroventricular delivery bypasses the BBB, enabling efficient cell homing to periventricular and hippocampal regions. Studies show that intracerebroventricularly delivered NSCs can migrate into the hippocampus, integrate into local circuits, and reduce inflammation and cell death [10, 52].

5.2 Intranasal delivery

Intranasal administration has emerged as a non-invasive and clinically feasible approach for NSC therapy. Cells delivered intranasally bypass the BBB by migrating through olfactory and trigeminal nerve pathways [53]. Intranasal delivery is suitable for repetitive dosing and acute settings such as post-CA care. Preclinical studies have demonstrated that intranasal-administered NSCs reach the hippocampus, reduce neuroinflammation, and improve functional outcomes [11, 22]. Moreover, this method avoids complications associated with surgical injection.

5.3 Intracranial delivery

Stereotactic injection of NSCs directly into infarcted or peri-infarct brain regions provides precise targeting of damaged tissue. This method allows for localized therapeutic effects and is often combined with biomaterial scaffolds to support graft survival and integration. However, IC delivery is highly invasive and may not be suitable for diffuse or acute injuries such as global ischemia or CA.

5.4 Intravenous and intra-arterial delivery

Systemic routes offer ease of administration but suffer from low targeting efficiency due to entrapment in peripheral organs like the lungs, liver, and spleen [54]. IA delivery, often through the carotid artery, can improve brain targeting but carries the risk of embolism and requires catheterization expertise [54]. Homing efficiency may be enhanced by preconditioning NSCs or modifying surface molecules to increase responsiveness to chemotactic signals.

5.5 Comparative analysis and optimization

Intracerebroventricular delivery may achieve higher initial retention in the ventricles and periventricular zones, whereas intranasal delivery offers better safety, repeatability, and scalability for clinical use. Advanced imaging modalities such as MRI and bioluminescence can be employed to monitor cell distribution and survival in vivo.

In addition to route selection, delivery parameters such as cell dose, suspension medium, injection rate, and timing relative to injury onset are critical for optimizing outcomes. Combination strategies, including intranasal delivery followed by biomaterial-supported intracranial injections, may further enhance efficacy. Ultimately, the choice of delivery method should be guided by the injury model, therapeutic goals, and clinical context. Tailoring delivery strategies to specific pathological conditions is essential to maximize the therapeutic potential of NSC-based interventions.

6. Enhancement of NSC therapy via cell modification

Despite the therapeutic promise of NSC transplantation, several challenges limit its efficacy in ischemic brain injury. These include low graft survival, limited integration into host circuitry, inadequate differentiation, and reduced responsiveness in the hostile ischemic microenvironment. To overcome these obstacles, multiple bioengineering strategies have been developed to enhance the functional properties and therapeutic potential of NSCs. **Table 1** provides a comparative overview of the strategies developed to enhance the efficacy of stem cell therapy.

6.1 MGE

MGE is an emerging biotechnology platform that enables the targeted remodeling of cell surface glycoconjugates—complex carbohydrates covalently attached to proteins and lipids—without the need for genetic modification. Originally developed to study glycan function, MGE has since evolved into a powerful method for enhancing cellular behavior and therapeutic efficacy in regenerative medicine. In the context of NSCs, this strategy has been employed to improve cell adhesion, viability, differentiation, and interactions with the ECM—all critical features for successful brain repair [11, 44].

MGE is a powerful technique that involves the biosynthetic incorporation of chemically modified monosaccharides into cell-surface glycans. The cell surface glycocalyx plays a fundamental role in mediating adhesion, migration, and intercellular signaling [44, 55]. This modification introduces thiol groups that enhance integrin-mediated adhesion, migration, and interaction with extracellular matrix components.

Among the most promising glycoengineering tools is Ac5ManNTProp, a thiol-modified N-acetylmannosamine analog [44, 55]. When metabolized by cells, Ac5ManNTProp is incorporated into sialic acid biosynthesis pathways and displayed on the cell surface as thiol-modified sialosides. This modification introduces reactive thiol groups to the cell membrane, enhancing interactions with ECM proteins such as laminin (see **Figure 1** for representative adhesion assay data) [44].

Importantly, Ac5ManNTProp-treated NSCs demonstrate significantly improved functional outcomes in animal models of cerebral ischemia [11]. Studies show better cell retention, survival, differentiation, and a notable reduction in neuroinflammation. These cells also appear to activate Wnt/β-catenin signaling, a pathway crucial for neural development, synaptic plasticity, and tissue repair [11].

6.2 Genetic modification

NSCs can be genetically engineered to overexpress genes that improve cell survival, promote neurogenesis, or enhance anti-inflammatory effects. Common targets include BDNF, GDNF, IL-10, and anti-apoptotic factors like Bcl-2 [30, 56, 57]. CRISPR/Cas9 [58] and viral vector systems [59] are used to introduce stable gene expression. These modifications can increase the efficacy of NSCs in reducing infarct

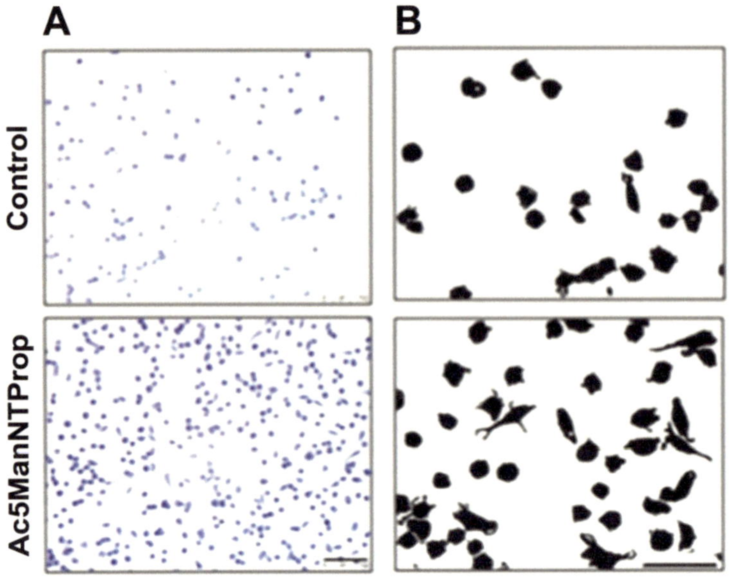

Figure 1.
Enhanced adhesion of glycoengineered NSCs to laminin (adapted from Du et al. [44]). Attachment (A) and morphology (B) of NSCs on laminin-coated surfaces with or without Ac5ManNTProp treatment. (A) Morphology of NSCs on laminin-coated ECM surfaces visualized by crystal violet staining. (B) Higher-magnification images showing the detailed morphology of adherent NSCs, demonstrating enhanced attachment and cell spreading in the Ac5ManNTProp-treated group on laminin surfaces. Scale bars: 50 μm.

volume and promoting behavioral recovery. However, safety concerns related to insertional mutagenesis and long-term gene expression need careful consideration.

6.3 Preconditioning strategies

Exposing NSCs to sub-lethal stressors such as hypoxia, inflammatory cytokines, or oxidative agents can 'precondition' them to better withstand the ischemic environment. Hypoxic preconditioning, for instance, upregulates hypoxia-inducible factors and anti-oxidant defenses, enhancing cell viability after transplantation [60, 61]. This approach also boosts the secretion of protective cytokines and promotes mitochondrial fitness.

6.4 Biomaterial encapsulation

Encapsulating NSCs in biocompatible hydrogels or scaffolds supports cell viability, improves engraftment, and provides a controlled release of trophic factors [61]. Commonly used materials include hyaluronic acid, collagen, and hydrogels. These scaffolds can be engineered to release chemokines or provide mechanical cues that favor neuronal differentiation. Biomaterials also act as physical barriers that shield grafts from host immune responses and oxidative damage.

6.5 Extracellular vesicle augmentation

NSCs naturally secrete EVs, including exosomes and microvesicles, that carry a diverse cargo of proteins, lipids, and RNAs [50]. EVs mediate many of the therapeutic effects attributed to NSCs and can be used independently or in combination with cell transplantation. Engineering NSCs to overexpress specific miRNAs or loading EVs with anti-inflammatory agents enhances their potency. EVs offer a cell-free alternative that reduces immunogenicity and simplifies storage and regulatory concerns.

In summary, the choice of enhancement strategy should be guided by the specific goals of therapy, the timing of intervention, and the characteristics of the target population. For example, in neonatal HIE, strategies that promote oligodendrocyte maturation and myelination may be prioritized, while in adult stroke, enhancing synaptic integration and angiogenesis may be more beneficial. Looking ahead, the development of enhanced NSC products with improved survival, targeting, and potency will be essential for the successful translation of stem cell therapy in cerebral ischemia. Rigorous preclinical validation and adherence to good manufacturing practice manufacturing standards will ensure safety and reproducibility in clinical applications.

7. In vitro and In vivo preclinical evidence

A growing body of preclinical evidence supports the efficacy of NSC therapy in various models of cerebral ischemia. These studies provide mechanistic insights and help establish the safety, optimal delivery conditions, and functional outcomes of different NSC formulations.

7.1 In vitro studies

In vitro assays have been pivotal in characterizing the neuroprotective effects of NSCs and evaluating enhancement strategies. NSCs exposed to oxygen-glucose deprivation (in vitro OGD model) mimic ischemic injury and allow quantification of cell survival, mitochondrial activity, and apoptosis markers.

Co-culture of NSCs with primary neurons or glial cells enables assessment of bystander effects, including anti-inflammatory signaling and promotion of neuronal outgrowth [22]. NSCs treated with MGE demonstrate improved adhesion to ECM substrate [45], enhanced cell viability and boosted ability of neuronal differentiation [11].

7.2 In vivo stroke models

In rodent MCAO models, NSC transplantation has been shown to reduce infarct volume, enhance neurogenesis, and improve behavioral performance [37, 38]. Enhanced NSCs, particularly those treated with preconditioning strategies, exhibit greater migration to the peri-infarct region, improved neuronal differentiation, and longer survival. These cells modulate the post-stroke microenvironment by reducing inflammation and supporting endogenous progenitors [51].

7.3 In vivo CA-induced ischemia model

In global cerebral ischemia models following CA, intranasally or Intracerebroventricular-delivered NSCs preferentially migrated to the hippocampus. These cells reduce microglial and astrocytic activation, restore synaptic density, and increase EEG quality indices such as EEG-IQ [10, 11].

Behavioral improvements include enhanced performance in memory tasks and reduced anxiety-like behavior. MGE-enhanced NSCs demonstrate superior migration toward hippocampal regions (see **Figure 2**) and greater suppression of gliosis compared to unmodified cells [11].

7.4 In vivo neonatal HIE model

In neonatal HIE models, NSCs contribute to white matter repair and promote oligodendrocyte lineage progression [42, 43].

Stem cell-derived extracellular vesicles have been reported to mitigate ischemic injury by delivering factors with neuroprotective, regenerative, and anti-inflammatory properties in neonatal ischemic brain [62]. These effects are particularly important for mitigating long-term deficits in infants with perinatal asphyxia.

7.5 Histological and molecular outcomes

NSC treatment across models results in reduced neuronal apoptosis (TUNEL, cleaved caspase-3), [63], increased neurogenesis (DCX, NeuN) [10], enhanced angiogenesis (CD31, VEGF), and upregulated synaptic markers (synapsin-1, PSD95) [11]. Transcriptomic and proteomic analyses reveal restoration of neurodevelopmental pathways and suppression of inflammatory cascades [64].

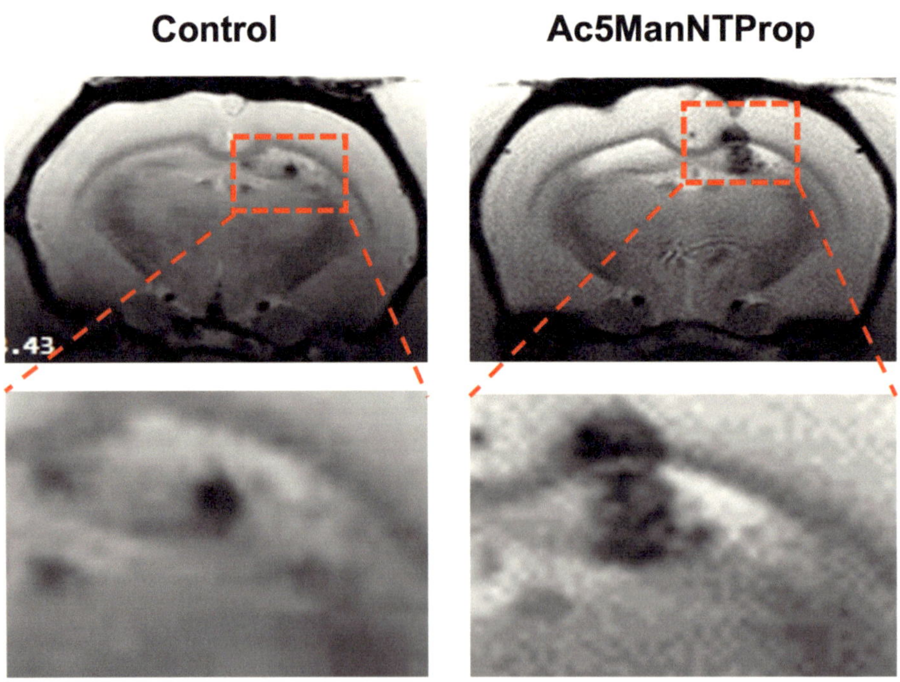

Figure 2.
Tracking glycoengineered NSCs in the brain via MRI (adapted from Du et al. [11]). Representative MRI images showing the localization of transplanted NSCs in a rat model of CA-induced ischemic brain injury, 30 days post-treatment. Left: animals treated with unmodified NSCs. Right: animals treated with Ac5ManNTProp-modified NSCs. Red boxes indicate regions of interest (hippocampus) showing hypointense signals corresponding to iron-labeled transplanted cells. Magnified views of these regions (bottom panels) highlight enhanced retention and signal intensity in the Ac5ManNTProp group, suggesting improved engraftment and survival.

7.6 Biodistribution and tracking

Advanced imaging techniques, including fluorescent tracking and MRI with superparamagnetic iron oxide (SPIO) labeling, confirm NSC migration to injury sites and provide longitudinal data on graft survival. These tools are essential for optimizing delivery protocols and confirming targeting accuracy.

7.6.1 Fluorescent tracking

Several approaches have been employed to trace transplanted NSCs. In one method, NSCs were pre-labeled with PKH26, a red fluorescent dye commonly used as a cell tracer; following intracerebroventricular delivery after CA-induced ischemic brain injury, PKH26-positive NSCs were mainly detected in the hippocampal CA1 region and cerebral cortex at 28 days post-transplantation [41]. Alternatively, other studies identified grafted human NSCs using the human nuclei marker Ku-86. Within 72 hours of Intracerebroventricular administration, Ku-86-positive cells were observed to migrate and localize primarily to the hippocampus in rats underwent asphyxia CA [10]. The markers, human mitochondria and MAP2 were also employed to visualize the migration and neuronal differentiation of transplanted human NSCs. MGE-modified NSCs effectively migrated to ischemic hippocampus and differentiate into functional mature neurons [11].

7.6.2 MRI with SPIO labeling

To evaluate whether MGE-modified NSCs exhibit enhanced homing capabilities in the brain following cerebral ischemia, both naïve and modified cells were labeled with Molday ION Rhodamine B (MIRB). These MIRB-labeled cells were subsequently introduced into the brain post-CA. Their presence was then identified as hypointense signals on T2-weighted MRI scans, allowing researchers to track the migration and localization of the NSCs with precision. One month after transplantation, the hypointense signal was more pronounced in the rat treated with glycoengineered NSCs compared to those with naïve NSCs [11] (See **Figure 2** for representative MRI images).

Collectively, these in vitro and in vivo studies establish a strong foundation for the therapeutic application of NSCs in cerebral ischemia. The results underscore the importance of cell enhancement strategies, precise delivery, and injury-specific tailoring to maximize efficacy and safety.

8. Clinical translation and future directions

The successful clinical translation of NSC therapy for cerebral ischemia requires careful consideration of multiple factors, including product standardization, regulatory approval, manufacturing scalability, delivery feasibility, and long-term safety monitoring. Although preclinical data have demonstrated consistent benefits across models of stroke, CA, and neonatal HIE, translating these findings into human studies poses both opportunities and challenges.

- Early-phase clinical trials: Some early-phase clinical trials have tested NSC-based therapies in patients with chronic stroke [65, 66]. These studies generally demonstrate safety and feasibility, with some reporting modest functional improvements. However, most trials have utilized unmodified cells and direct intracerebral delivery. Lessons from these studies underscore the need for improved delivery routes, enhanced cell formulations, and better-defined patient selection criteria.

- Timing and patient stratification: The therapeutic window for NSC therapy is likely to vary by condition. For ischemic stroke, early delivery may offer the best opportunity to mitigate secondary damage and promote repair. In post-CA patients, interventions must be compatible with ICU care, non-invasive, and rapidly deployable. In neonates with HIE, early identification and combination with hypothermia may yield the highest benefit. Stratification based on injury severity, age, comorbidities, and genetic background may also help personalize treatment and improve outcomes.

- Manufacturing and regulatory considerations: Scaling up NSC production requires adherence to good manufacturing practices (GMP), rigorous quality control, and reproducibility across batches. Key release criteria include viability, identity (e.g., Nestin, Sox2), purity, sterility, and potency (e.g., neurotrophic factor secretion or neurite outgrowth assays). Enhanced NSCs—via MGE, gene editing, or biomaterial encapsulation—will require additional safety testing to rule out tumorigenicity, off-target effects, and immunogenicity.

- Ethical and logistical challenges: Autologous NSC therapies offer immunologic advantages but face delays in production and variable quality depending on donor health. Allogeneic 'off-the-shelf' products provide scalability but raise concerns about immune rejection and the need for immunosuppression. Strategies to balance efficacy, accessibility, and safety will shape the design of future clinical programs.

- Integration with rehabilitation and adjunct therapies: Stem cell-based interventions are unlikely to be curative alone. Combining NSC transplantation with physical rehabilitation, neuromodulation, and pharmacologic neuroprotectants may offer synergistic effects.

- Future research directions: Key areas for future investigation include: (1) identification of optimal biomarkers for patient selection and response tracking; (2) evaluation of repeated or staged dosing; (3) expansion to large-animal and primate models with functional imaging and electrophysiology; and (4) long-term safety and efficacy monitoring.

In conclusion, while the path to clinical adoption of NSC therapy for cerebral ischemia remains complex, advances in stem cell engineering, delivery science, and clinical trial design have significantly accelerated progress. With continued multidisciplinary collaboration and translational rigor, NSC-based interventions hold strong potential to redefine the therapeutic landscape for ischemic stroke, CA-induced global ischemia, and neonatal brain injury.

DOI: http://dx.doi.org/10.5772/intechopen.1012582

Author details

Xiao Liu
Department of Neurosurgery, University of Maryland School of Medicine, Baltimore, MD, USA

*Address all correspondence to: akcl.whu@outlook.com; xiao.liu@som.umaryland.edu

References

[1] Lee RHC et al. Cerebral ischemia and neuroregeneration. Neural Regeneration Research. 2018;**13**(3):373-385

[2] Sasannia S et al. Blood-brain barrier breakdown in brain ischemia: Insights from MRI perfusion imaging. Neurotherapeutics. 2025;**22**(1):e00516

[3] Aboobacker IM et al. Life after stroke from survivors perspective: A descriptive cross-sectional study. Clinical Epidemiology and Global Health. 2025;**33**:102001

[4] Chan PS et al. Long-term outcomes among elderly survivors of out-of-hospital cardiac arrest. Journal of the American Heart Association. 2016;**5**(3):e002924

[5] Chan PS et al. Long-term outcomes in elderly survivors of in-hospital cardiac arrest. The New England Journal of Medicine. 2013;**368**(11):1019-1026

[6] Warenits AM et al. Motor cortex and hippocampus display decreased Heme oxygenase activity 2 weeks after ventricular fibrillation cardiac arrest in rats. Frontiers in Medicine (Lausanne). 2020;**7**:513

[7] Halpin S et al. Long-term neuropsychological and behavioral outcome of mild and moderate hypoxic ischemic encephalopathy. Early Human Development. 2022;**165**:105541

[8] Zhao L et al. Neural stem cell therapy for brain disease. World Journal of Stem Cells. 2021;**13**(9):1278-1292

[9] Ottoboni L, von Wunster B, Martino G. Therapeutic plasticity of neural stem cells. Frontiers in Neurology. 2020;**11**:148

[10] Wang Z et al. Intracerebroventricular administration of hNSCs improves neurological recovery after cardiac arrest in rats. Stem Cell Reviews and Reports. 2021;**17**(3):923-937

[11] Du J et al. Metabolically glycoengineered neural stem cells boost neural repair after cardiac arrest. Advanced Functional Materials. 2024;**34**(17):2309866

[12] Rehman S et al. Molecular mechanisms of ischemic stroke: A review integrating clinical imaging and therapeutic perspectives. Biomedicine. 2024;**12**(4):812. DOI: 10.3390/biomedicines12040812

[13] Neumar RW. Molecular mechanisms of ischemic neuronal injury. Annals of Emergency Medicine. 2000;**36**(5):483-506

[14] Kuriakose D, Xiao Z. Patho-physiology and treatment of stroke: Present status and future perspectives. International Journal of Molecular Sciences. 2020;**21**(20):7609. DOI: 10.3390/ijms21207609

[15] Levinson S, Pulli B, Heit JJ. Neuroinflammation and acute ischemic stroke: Impact on translational research and clinical care. Frontiers in Surgery. 2025;**12**:1501359

[16] Chen W et al. Astrogliosis and glial scar in ischemic stroke—focused on mechanism and treatment. Experimental Neurology. 2025;**385**:115131

[17] Conti E et al. A novel model of light-induced middle cerebral artery occlusion and recanalization in mice. Communications Biology. 2025;**8**(1):1117

[18] Knezic A et al. Optimising the photothrombotic model of stroke in the C57BI/6 and FVB/N strains of mouse. Scientific Reports. 2022;**12**(1):7598

[19] Bazzigaluppi P et al. Frequency selective neuronal modulation triggers spreading depolarizations in the rat endothelin-1 model of stroke. Journal of Cerebral Blood Flow and Metabolism. 2021;**41**(10):2756-2768

[20] Jia X et al. Early electrophysiologic markers predict functional outcome associated with temperature manipulation after cardiac arrest in rats. Critical Care Medicine. 2008;**36**(6):1909-1916

[21] Jia X, Liu X. Stem cell therapy after neurological injuries. In: Haider KH, editor. Handbook of Stem Cell Applications. Singapore: Springer Nature Singapore; 2023. pp. 1-28

[22] Wang Z et al. Neuroprotection of NSC therapy is superior to Glibenclamide in cardiac arrest-induced brain injury via neuroinflammation regulation. Translational Stroke Research. 2023;**14**(5):723-739

[23] Dave KR et al. Ventricular fibrillation-induced cardiac arrest in the rat as a model of global cerebral ischemia. Translational Stroke Research. 2013;**4**(5):571-578

[24] Liu H et al. Novel modification of potassium chloride induced cardiac arrest model for aged mice. Aging and Disease. 2018;**9**(1):31-39

[25] Ourednik J et al. Protocol to optimize the Rice-Vannucci rat pup model of perinatal asphyxia to ensure predictable hypoxic-ischemic cerebral lesions. STAR Protocols. 2024;**5**(2):103025

[26] Recker R et al. Rodent neonatal bilateral carotid artery occlusion with hypoxia mimics human hypoxic-ischemic injury. Journal of Cerebral Blood Flow and Metabolism. 2009;**29**(7):1305-1316

[27] Wilson MD. Animal models of cerebral palsy: Hypoxic brain injury in the newborn. Iranian Journal of Child Neurology. 2015;**9**(2):9-16

[28] Cai Z et al. Chronic ischemia preferentially causes white matter injury in the neonatal rat brain. Brain Research. 2001;**898**(1):126-135

[29] Liu X, Jia X. Neuroprotection of stem cells against ischemic brain injury: From bench to clinic. Translational Stroke Research. 2024;**15**(4):691-713

[30] Dause TJ et al. The neural stem cell secretome across neurodevelopment. Experimental Neurology. 2022;**355**:114142

[31] Zhou G et al. Potential mechanisms and perspectives in ischemic stroke treatment using stem cell therapies. Frontiers in Cell and Developmental Biology. 2021;**9**:646927. DOI: 10.3389/fcell.2021.646927

[32] Santos MFD, Roxo C, Solá S. Oxidative-signaling in neural stem cell-mediated plasticity: Implications for neurodegenerative diseases. Antioxidants (Basel). 2021;**10**(7):1088. DOI: 10.3390/antiox10071088

[33] Imitola J et al. Directed migration of neural stem cells to sites of CNS injury by the stromal cell-derived factor 1alpha/CXC chemokine receptor 4 pathway. Proceedings of the National Academy of Sciences of the United States of America. 2004;**101**(52):18117-18122

[34] Belmadani A et al. Chemokines regulate the migration of neural progenitors to sites of neuroinflammation. Journal of Neuroscience. 2006;**26**(12):3182-3191

[35] Takeuchi H et al. Intravenously transplanted human neural stem cells migrate to the injured spinal cord in adult mice in an SDF-1-and HGF-dependent manner. Neuroscience Letters. 2007;**426**(2):69-74

[36] Palma-Tortosa S et al. Neuronal replacement in stem cell therapy for stroke: Filling the gap. Frontiers in Cell and Developmental Biology. 2021;**9**:662636. DOI: 10.3389/fcell.2021.662636

[37] Jin K et al. Effect of human neural precursor cell transplantation on endogenous neurogenesis after focal cerebral ischemia in the rat. Brain Research. 2011;**1374**:56-62

[38] Ryu S et al. Human neural stem cells promote proliferation of endogenous neural stem cells and enhance angiogenesis in ischemic rat brain. Neural Regeneration Research. 2016;**11**(2):298-304

[39] Andres RH et al. Human neural stem cells enhance structural plasticity and axonal transport in the ischaemic brain. Brain. 2011;**134**(Pt 6):1777-1789

[40] Watanabe T et al. A human neural stem cell line provides neuroprotection and improves neurological performance by early intervention of neuroinflammatory system. Brain Research. 2016;**1631**:194-203

[41] Wang Z et al. Intracerebroventricular administration of neural stem cells after cardiac arrest. Annual International Conference of the IEEE Engineering in Medicine and Biology Society. 2019;**2019**:4213-4216

[42] van Velthoven CT et al. Mesenchymal stem cell treatment after neonatal hypoxic-ischemic brain injury improves behavioral outcome and induces neuronal and oligodendrocyte regeneration. Brain, Behavior, and Immunity. 2010;**24**(3):387-393

[43] Bennet L et al. Cell therapy for neonatal hypoxia-ischemia and cerebral palsy. Annals of Neurology. 2012;**71**(5):589-600

[44] Du J et al. Glycoengineering human neural stem cells (hNSCs) for adhesion improvement using a novel thiol-modified N-acetylmannosamine (ManNAc) analog. Biomaterials Advances. 2022;**134**:112675

[45] Du J et al. Glycoengineering human neural and adipose stem cells with novel thiol-modified N-Acetylmannosamine (ManNAc) analogs. Cells. 2021;**10**(2):377. DOI: 10.3390/cells10020377

[46] Tang X et al. Advances in genetically modified neural stem cell therapy for central nervous system injury and neurological diseases. Stem Cell Research & Therapy. 2024;**15**(1):482

[47] Liang Y, Walczak P, Bulte JW. The survival of engrafted neural stem cells within hyaluronic acid hydrogels. Biomaterials. 2013;**34**(22):5521-5529

[48] Cao H et al. Current hydrogel advances in physicochemical and biological response-driven biomedical application diversity. Signal Transduction and Targeted Therapy. 2021;**6**(1):426

[49] Zhang T et al. Adjudin-preconditioned neural stem cells enhance neuroprotection after ischemia reperfusion in mice. Stem Cell Research & Therapy. 2017;**8**(1):248

[50] Wang J et al. Human neural stem cell–derived extracellular vesicles protect against ischemic stroke by activating the PI3K/AKT/mTOR pathway. Neural Regeneration Research. 2025;**20**(11):3245-3258. DOI: 10.4103/NRR.NRR-D-23-01144

[51] Othman FA, Tan SC. Preconditioning strategies to enhance neural stem cell-based therapy for ischemic stroke. Brain Sciences. 2020;**10**(11):893

[52] Zhang M et al. Comparative outcomes of intravenous, intranasal, and

Intracerebroventricular transplantation of human neural stem cells in mice model of ischemic stroke. Current Stem Cell Research and Therapy. 2025;**20**(2):183-198

[53] Liu X, Jia X. Stem cell therapy for ischemic brain injury: Early intranasal delivery after cardiac arrest. Translational Stroke Research. 2024;**15**(3):495-497

[54] Zhang S et al. Optimizing stem cell therapy after ischemic brain injury. Journal of Stroke. 2020;**22**(3):286

[55] Du J et al. Improving Schwann cell differentiation from human adipose stem cells with metabolic glycoengineering. Cells. 2023;**12**(8):1190

[56] Mooney R et al. Bcl-2 overexpression improves survival and efficacy of neural stem cell-mediated enzyme prodrug therapy. Stem Cells International. 2018;**2018**:7047496

[57] Yang J et al. Adult neural stem cells expressing IL-10 confer potent immunomodulation and remyelination in experimental autoimmune encephalitis. The Journal of Clinical Investigation. 2009;**119**(12):3678-3691

[58] Bressan RB et al. Efficient CRISPR/Cas9-assisted gene targeting enables rapid and precise genetic manipulation of mammalian neural stem cells. Development. 2017;**144**(4):635-648

[59] Asmamaw, Mengstie M. Viral vectors for the in vivo delivery of CRISPR components: Advances and challenges. Frontiers in Bioengineering and Biotechnology. 2022;**10**:895713. DOI: 10.3389/fbioe.2022.895713

[60] Theus MH et al. In vitro hypoxic preconditioning of embryonic stem cells as a strategy of promoting cell survival and functional benefits after transplantation into the ischemic rat brain. Experimental Neurology. 2008;**210**(2):656-670

[61] Chacko SM et al. Hypoxic preconditioning induces the expression of prosurvival and proangiogenic markers in mesenchymal stem cells. American Journal of Physiology. Cell Physiology. 2010;**299**(6):C1562-C1570

[62] Nguyen NP et al. Brain tissue-derived extracellular vesicle mediated therapy in the neonatal ischemic brain. International Journal of Molecular Sciences. 2022;**23**(2):620. DOI: 10.3390/ijms23020620

[63] Wang L et al. Mild hypothermia combined with neural stem cell transplantation for hypoxic-ischemic encephalopathy: Neuroprotective effects of combined therapy. Neural Regeneration Research. 2014;**9**(19):1745-1752. DOI: 10.4103/1673-5374.143417

[64] Hur H-J et al. Conditioned medium of human pluripotent stem cell-derived neural precursor cells exerts neurorestorative effects against ischemic stroke model. International Journal of Molecular Sciences. 2022;**23**(14):7787

[65] Kalladka D et al. Human neural stem cells in patients with chronic ischaemic stroke (PISCES): A phase 1, first-in-man study. Lancet. 2016;**388**(10046):787-796

[66] Qiao LY et al. A two-year follow-up study of cotransplantation with neural stem/progenitor cells and mesenchymal stromal cells in ischemic stroke patients. Cell Transplantation. 2014;**23**(Suppl. 1):S65-S72

Section 2

Brain Development

Chapter 3

Microphysiological Systems: Advancing Insights into Brain Development and Disorders

Farjana Yasmin, Rodrigo Cristofoletti and Janny Piñeiro-Llanes

Abstract

Cerebral organoids have transformed neuroscience, replicating key features of brain development to study neurodevelopmental, neuropsychiatric and neurodegenerative disorders. These models offer critical insights into human-specific processes and have been further enhanced by technologies like brain-on-a-chip platforms and multi-organ systems, enabling systemic disease modeling and advancing drug discovery. This chapter explores brain development from conception to adulthood, highlighting how microphysiological systems model healthy and diseased states. It begins by outlining neurodevelopmental milestones such as neural induction, progenitor differentiation, synaptic formation, and neuroplasticity as the brain evolves through childhood, adolescence, and adulthood. These processes establish the foundation for understanding disruptions leading to disorders. Brain organoids are emphasized as groundbreaking tools, offering unparalleled fidelity in studying conditions like Down's syndrome, Leigh's syndrome, autism spectrum disorders, and Alzheimer's disease. These models address critical gaps in neuroscience, driving advances in drug discovery and therapeutic innovation. Emerging technologies, including microfluidic platforms, gene editing, and machine learning, expand the scope of organoid research, enabling investigations into complex interactions and biocomputing applications. Despite their promise, challenges in functional maturity, scalability, and ethical considerations persist. Overcoming these barriers will further enhance brain organoid research, paving the way for deeper insights into brain development and innovative treatments for neurological disorders.

Keywords: cerebral organoids, neurodevelopment, microphysiological models, disease modeling, precision medicine, therapeutic applications

1. Introduction

Understanding brain development is fundamental to advancing neurological health. Investigating the processes of brain growth, function, and adaptability reveals critical periods for cognitive and emotional maturation. This knowledge enables early interventions for neurodevelopmental disorders, such as autism spectrum disorder (ASD) and attention-deficit/hyperactivity disorder (ADHD). Additionally, understanding brain maturation and neuroplasticity informs the development of targeted therapies for neurological conditions, including epilepsy, stroke, and neurodegenerative diseases.

In vitro cell cultures are essential research tools for modeling human development and diseases. However, traditional two-dimensional (2D) models often lack the structural and functional complexity required to replicate *in vivo* conditions accurately. To address these limitations, microphysiological systems (MPS) have emerged as transformative technologies in biomedical research. These systems encompass a range of advanced models, including static organoids and dynamic organ-on-chip platforms, which aim to emulate the architecture, functionality, and physiological environment of human tissues and organs.

Organoids, one of the most prominent examples of static MPS, are three-dimensional (3D) cell clusters that self-organize and differentiate into functional cell types. *In vitro* organoids replicate key structural and functional features of their *in vivo* counterparts, making them highly relevant for studying human organ development and disease pathogenesis. Organoids can be engineered from embryonic stem cells (ESCs), induced pluripotent stem cells (iPSCs), or neonatal or adult stem cells (ASCs) [1, 2]. They provide a powerful tool for modeling cellular diversity, tissue architecture, and developmental processes of a certain organ, with significant translational potential in regenerative medicine, drug discovery, and precision medicine [3].

Dynamic MPS, such as organ-on-chip systems, extend the capabilities of static models by incorporating mechanical and fluidic stimuli to simulate the dynamic physiological conditions of the human body. These systems utilize microfluidics and engineered scaffolds to replicate tissue-tissue interfaces, mechanical forces, and dynamic perfusion, thereby capturing the interactions between multiple organ systems. For brain research, neurovascular unit-on-chip models have been developed to study the blood-brain barrier, neuroinflammation, and the interplay between neurons, glial cells, and vascular components. Dynamic MPS complement static models by addressing limitations such as the absence of vascularization and functional integration in organoids.

Recent progress in human iPSC (hiPSC) technology has further enhanced the utility of MPS by enabling the generation of patient-specific models. These systems provide a scalable platform for studying human brain diseases. This approach is particularly valuable for investigating complex neurological disorders, such as ASD, schizophrenia, Alzheimer's disease (AD), and Parkinson's disease (PD), which often arise from heterogeneous combinations of genetic variants and environmental interactions. While the human brain is the ideal system for studying these conditions, its study is constrained by ethical considerations, limited tissue availability, and technical challenges associated with culturing brain tissue [4].

By bridging the gap between traditional *in vitro* methods and the complexities of human biology, MPS—both static and dynamic—offer unparalleled opportunities for elucidating the molecular mechanisms of brain development and disease. These advancements enable the exploration of novel therapeutic strategies and accelerate the translation of basic research into clinical applications.

This chapter explores the intricate stages of brain development and delves into how brain organoids replicate key features of this process, examining the technical approaches, applications, and challenges associated with organoid models. Topics include the use of organoids in disease research, regenerative medicine, and personalized therapies, as well as emerging innovations such as multiorgan systems and organoid intelligence. The chapter concludes with a discussion on future directions and key milestones, showcasing how organoid technology is transforming our understanding of brain development and advancing biomedical research.

2. Brain development from conception to adulthood

2.1 The stages of brain development

The human brain development starts around three weeks of gestation with the formation of the neural tube, which later closes to form the foundational structure of the central nervous system. By four weeks, major regions of the brain, the forebrain, midbrain, hindbrain, and optic vesicle, emerge in their primitive forms, laying the groundwork for later specialization. By six months of gestation, irregular ridges, or convolutions, begin to form, indicating the rapid growth and folding characteristic of the human brain.

The migration of neurons is critical for the organization of the brain and is particularly prominent in forming the cerebral cortex, a defining feature of primates, including humans. Neurons travel from their place of origin to their final destinations, guided by a complex interplay of molecular signals and environmental cues. Once neurons reach their final location, they establish functional connections through axons. Axons navigate through intricate pathways, ending their journey when they meet the branching areas called dendrites of other neurons. These connections form synapses, enabling electrical signals to transfer between cells. At the synapse, neurotransmitters allow for excitatory or inhibitory communication, supporting the specialized functions of neuronal networks [5].

Important structural maturation continues toward adolescence. During postnatal development, gray matter density follows a region-specific trajectory, peaking first

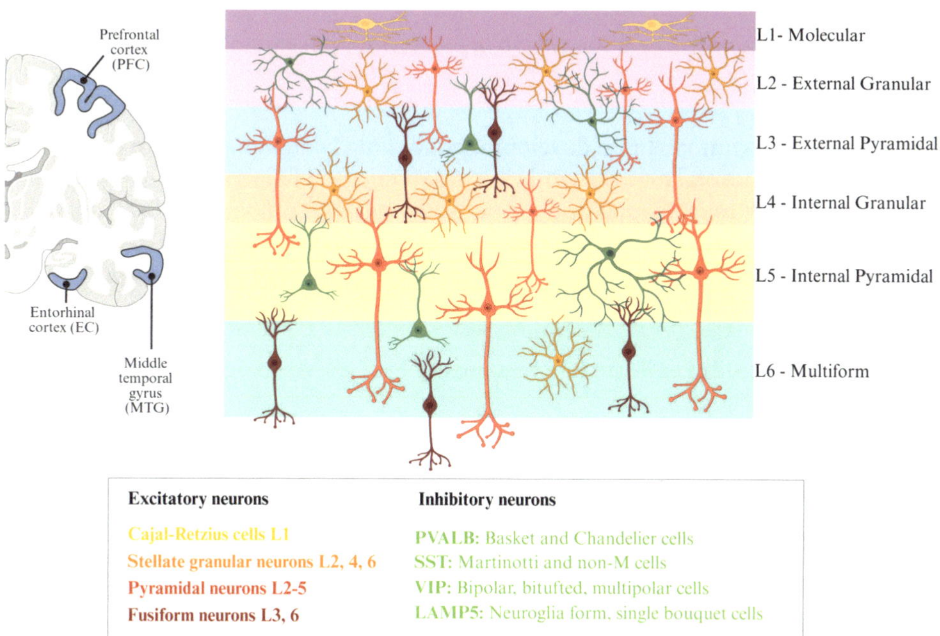

Figure 1.
Illustration of the diverse neuronal populations and their distribution across the six cortical layers of the human brain. Excitatory neurons (Cajal-Retzius cells, stellate granular neurons, pyramidal neurons, and fusiform neurons) and inhibitory neurons (basket and chandelier cells, Martinotti cells, bipolar cells, and others) are depicted within distinct cortical layers (L1–L6), emphasizing their unique roles in neural circuitry. The schematic highlights the structural complexity and specialized functions within the prefrontal cortex (PFC), entorhinal cortex (EC), and middle temporal gyrus (MTG), demonstrating the intricate organization of the human cortex. Created with BioRender.com.

in the sensorimotor cortex and later in the prefrontal cortex. Subcortical regions like the limbic and reward systems mature earlier, often leading to an imbalance between emotional regulation and cognitive control during adolescence. The prefrontal cortex, responsible for higher-order executive functions, gradually integrates with sensory and subcortical systems, supporting the development of complex behaviors and decision-making capabilities.

A hallmark of the human brain is its six-layered cortical architecture, a feature unique to humans and some primates. Each cortical layer (**Figure 1**), the molecular layer, external granular and pyramidal layers, internal granular and pyramidal layers, and the multiform layer, have specialized neurons with distinct roles in information processing and transmission. This multilayered design supports higher-order functions, such as movement, sensation, and cognition, distinguishing the human brain in evolutionary terms [6].

During adolescence, significant remodeling occurs within the cortex. Synaptic pruning, a process in which excess synapses formed during childhood are selectively eliminated, reshapes cortical circuitry. This dynamic remodeling enhances the efficiency of neural networks, supporting intellectual and emotional development. However, the high plasticity of the adolescent brain also increases its susceptibility to environmental influences, both beneficial and harmful [7].

Understanding the progression of brain development, from the migration of neurons to the maturation of cortical architecture, is essential for unraveling the mechanisms underlying neurological health and disorders.

3. Organoid technology: A revolutionary approach to studying brain development

Understanding human brain development has long been a challenge in neuroscience. Traditional animal models, while informative, often fail to replicate human-specific aspects of neurodevelopment due to interspecies differences. Cerebral organoids address this gap by emulating key aspects of early brain development. This model provides a scalable platform for studying neurodevelopment, disease mechanisms, and therapeutic interventions.

3.1 How do organoids replicate key features of human brain development?

Cerebral organoids replicate several key features of human brain development, such as neurogenesis, regional organization (including cortical layers), and synaptic activity. Among these, cortical cerebral organoids, specialized models of the cerebral cortex, stand out for their ability to mimic the layered architecture and cellular dynamics of this critical brain region. These models self-organize into structures that emulate the layered architecture of the cortex, making them highly relevant for studying human-specific neurodevelopmental processes [8, 9]. For example, cortical organoids have been used to model the development of the cerebral cortex, a region responsible for higher cognitive functions such as reasoning and memory [10].

The terminology surrounding these models has evolved to reflect their capabilities accurately. While the media and some scientific contexts often refer to them as "mini brains" or "brains in a dish," such descriptors can be misleading, particularly when discussing cortical organoids. These terms suggest a level of complexity and functionality that exceeds the current capabilities of these models. Using precise terms, such as

DOI: http://dx.doi.org/10.5772/intechopen.1011630

"cortical cerebral organoids," establishes realistic expectations and promotes accurate communication about their potential and limitations. Specifying the brain region represented, such as "cortical brain organoids," not only highlights their targeted focus but also avoids conflating them with broader cerebral organoids or overestimating the scope of current technology [11].

3.2 Regional specificity of cerebral organoids

Cortical brain organoids are derived from human pluripotent stem cells, including iPSCs. These cells are directed to differentiate into neural tissues through carefully orchestrated steps. In a groundbreaking study, Lancaster et al. [8] pioneered the creation of cerebral organoids by inducing iPSCs to form neuroectodermal tissues, providing the foundational methods that have since been refined [8]. Specifically, this

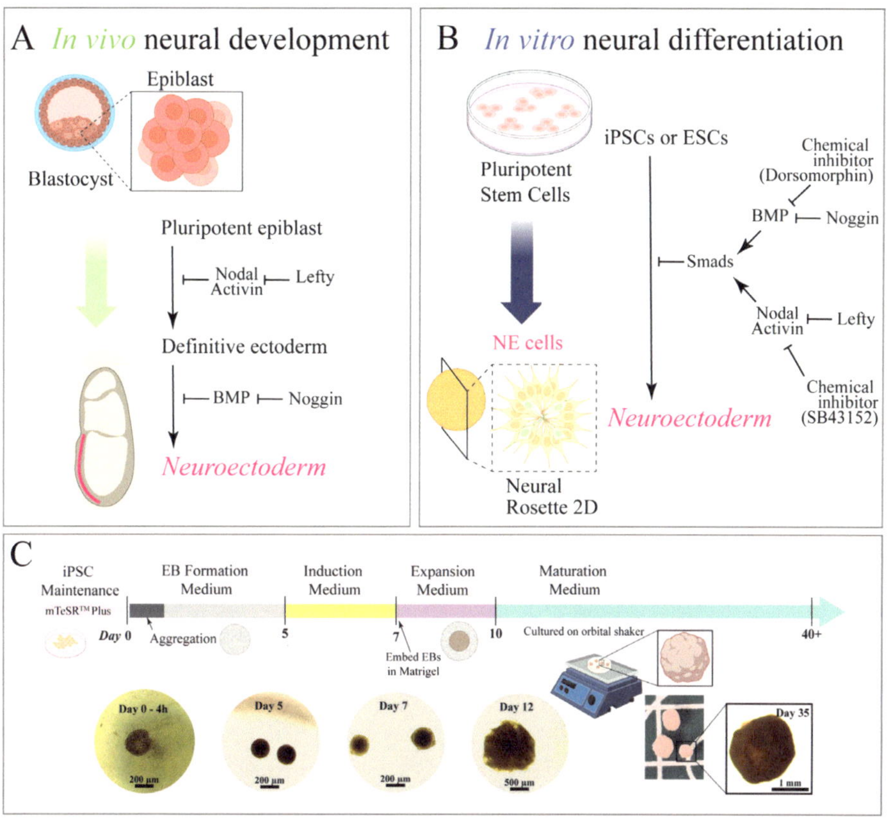

Figure 2.
In Vitro Neural Differentiation Mimics In Vivo Neural Development to Enable Cerebral Organoid Formation. (A) In vivo neural development: In the embryonic context, the pluripotent epiblast transitions into the neuroectoderm through molecular signals, including Nodal/Activin, BMP, and Noggin, orchestrating the formation of definitive ectoderm and subsequent neuroectoderm. (B) In vitro neural differentiation: Pluripotent stem cells (iPSCs or ESCs) recapitulate this process under defined conditions, with Nodal/Activin and BMP inhibition (via chemical inhibitors such as SB431542 and dorsomorphin) mimicking the molecular cues for neuroectoderm differentiation. The resulting neural epithelial (NE) cells form neural rosettes, a hallmark of neuroectoderm in vitro. (C) Cerebral organoid generation process: A stepwise protocol using a commercial kit from STEMcell Technologies begins with iPSC aggregation to form embryoid bodies (EBs). These are embedded in Matrigel and cultured on an orbital shaker to promote expansion and maturation, resulting in cerebral organoids with advanced structural and cellular complexity by day 35. Created with BioRender.com.

process involved the induction of iPSCs to neuroectodermal fates using dual-SMAD inhibition, which blocks the bone morphogenic protein (BMP) and the transforming growth factor beta (TGF-β) signaling pathways to suppress mesodermal and endodermal differentiation, effectively emulating early stages of neural induction (**Figures 2** and **3**). Then, iPSCs were aggregated into embryoid bodies and embedded in Matrigel, which provided extracellular matrix support. This approach, combined with bioreactors to enhance nutrient and oxygen distribution, enabled the formation of cortical-like structures that self-organized into layers resembling the developing human brain.

Subsequent advancements, such as those by Paşca et al. [9], refined protocols to generate region-specific organoids, including models of the forebrain, by supplementing cultures with signaling factors like wingless-related integration (WNT) agonists for forebrain specification and fibroblast growth factor (FGF) for midbrain development [9]. These methods have been instrumental in developing cortical organoids, which exhibit enhanced neural connectivity, cellular diversity, and features such as spontaneous electrical activity and synaptic formation, hallmarks of early neural circuitry [12]. These advancements have also enabled more detailed

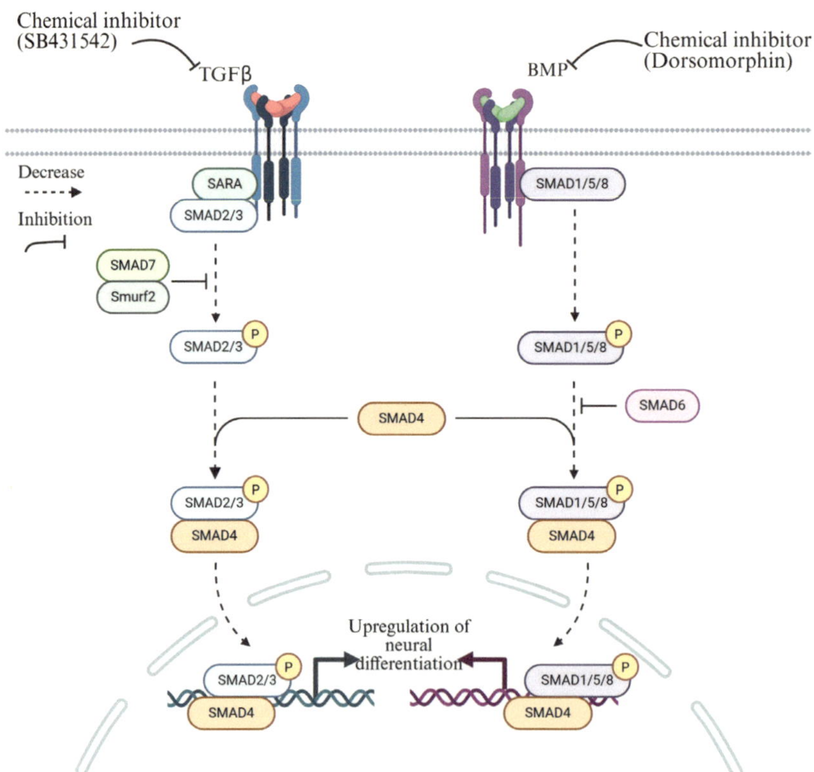

Figure 3.
Schematic representation of the dual SMAD inhibition pathway promoting neural differentiation. The TGF-β signaling pathway (left) and the BMP signaling pathway (right) are inhibited using chemical inhibitors SB431542 and dorsomorphin, respectively. SB431542 blocks TGF-β receptor activation, preventing the phosphorylation of SMAD2/3, while dorsomorphin inhibits BMP receptor activation, halting the phosphorylation of SMAD1/5/8. Both pathways converge on SMAD4, a critical co-SMAD involved in transcriptional regulation. The disruption of these pathways leads to a reduction in SMAD-mediated inhibitory signals, upregulating neural differentiation. This strategy is integral to the unguided protocol for generating cerebral organoids. Created with BioRender.com.

studies of synaptic activity and network formation, which were previously challenging to achieve in animal models.

Further protocol optimizations have enabled the generation of organoids representing a broad range of brain regions beyond the dorsal cortex, including the ganglionic eminence, striatum [13], hippocampus [14], pituitary gland [15], thalamus [16], midbrain [17], and cerebellum [18]. This expanded repertoire supports investigations into local and long-range neuronal interactions and regional specialization. Despite this diversity, cortical organoids remain central to modeling early cortical development and investigating diseases affecting this critical brain region.

3.3 Advantages and limitations compared to animal models

The advantages of cortical brain organoid technology over traditional animal models are substantial, although not without their own limitations. One major benefit is the ability to create human-specific models that reflect the complexity and diversity of human brain development. While animal models have provided important foundational knowledge, they often do not capture the unique aspects of human neurobiology. For example, certain human-specific protein variants, such as mutations in the *APP* (amyloid precursor protein) and *MAPT* (microtubule-associated protein tau) genes, are not present in most animal models [19]. These mutations lead to the characteristic amyloid plaques and tau tangles seen in Alzheimer's disease, which are critical to understanding human-specific neurodegenerative processes [20]. In contrast, organoids have successfully demonstrated key pathological features, including amyloid aggregation and tau hyperphosphorylation, providing insights about these diseases that were not achievable with rodent models [21].

Another key advantage of organoids is their ability to recapitulate the human-specific six-layered neocortical structure (**Figures 1** and **4**), a hallmark of human brain organization that is absent or rudimentary in most animal models. These six cortical layers, each with distinct cellular composition and connectivity, are critical for higher-order cognitive functions, such as sensory processing, language, and abstract reasoning. Recent studies demonstrate that cerebral organoids can develop these layered structures, with clear segregation of upper and deep cortical layers, resembling the architecture seen in the human fetal brain [22]. This capability provides a powerful platform to study the development and pathology of the human neocortex, which cannot be fully replicated in non-human models. Additionally, organoids are cost-effective because they are scalable and can be cultured in large quantities, making them an attractive option for high-throughput screening and personalized medicine applications [23].

However, limitations remain. Organoids lack vascularization, which restricts their maturation and functional integration. This limitation impacts their ability to model complex processes, such as blood-brain barrier development and long-range neuronal connectivity. Moreover, organoids typically display a necrotic core due to limited oxygen and nutrient diffusion, a challenge that hinders their maturation. Additionally, the process of generating organoids and allowing them to mature takes several months, which limits their use in certain applications, such as rapid drug testing or disease modeling at various stages of development [24]. Efforts to address these challenges, such as vascularized organoids and integration with microfluidic systems, represent promising directions for enhancing organoid functionality. By bridging the gap between in vitro and in vivo models, cerebral organoids hold the potential to unravel fundamental questions about human brain development and to inform the development of targeted therapies for neurological disorders.

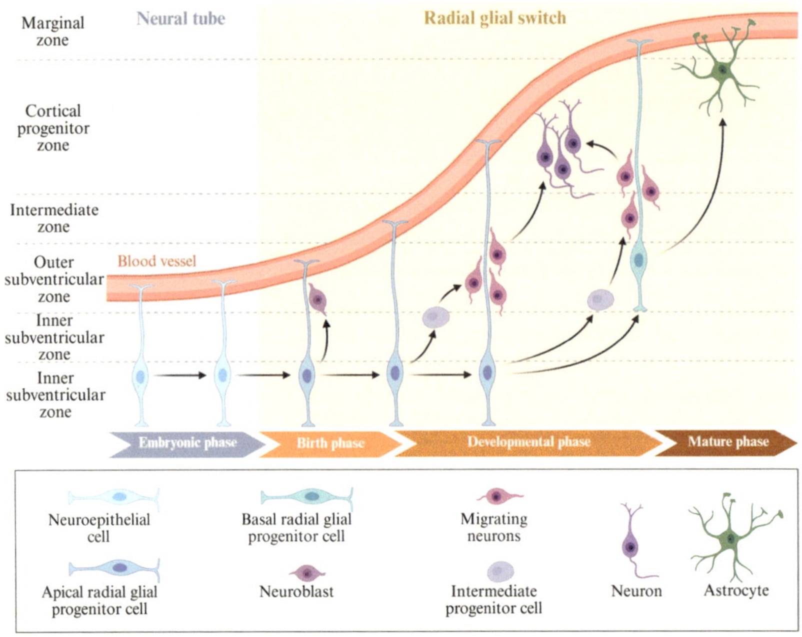

Figure 4.
Illustration of the cortical development of astrocytes within transient developmental zones of the evolving human cortex. Notably, the subventricular zone (SVZ) in the human brain is distinctly partitioned into inner and outer regions, a structural organization absent in mouse models. Additionally, the human cortical plate (CP) undergoes complex maturation into a six-layered structure, a defining characteristic differentiating human cortical organization from the simpler mouse counterpart. These unique developmental patterns highlight species-specific adaptations in astrocyte emergence and cortical architecture. Created with BioRender.com.

4. Organoid models of brain development

As previously discussed, cerebral organoids are derived from pluripotent stem cells, such as iPSCs or ESCs, and can be generated using either guided or unguided differentiation protocols. These methods allow for the modeling of distinct aspects of brain development and the uncovering of mechanisms underlying human neurodevelopmental processes.

4.1 Overview of guided and unguided approaches

4.1.1 Unguided differentiation protocols

Unguided differentiation protocols harness the intrinsic self-organizing potential of pluripotent stem cells to form neural tissues. The process typically begins with the formation of embryoid bodies (EBs), spherical aggregates of stem cells. Dual-SMAD inhibition promotes neuroectodermal differentiation by suppressing mesodermal and endodermal pathways through inhibition of BMP and TGF-β signaling (**Figures 2** and **3**). Neuroepithelial aggregates are then embedded in ECM scaffolds, such as Matrigel, to provide structural support. Dynamic culture systems, including spinning bioreactors or orbital shakers, enhance nutrient and oxygen diffusion, facilitating the development of cortical-like regions with radial glial scaffolds and progenitor zone [8].

DOI: http://dx.doi.org/10.5772/intechopen.1011630

4.1.2 Guided differentiation protocols

Guided protocols use specific exogenous factors to direct stem cell fate toward desired brain regions. For instance, forebrain organoids are generated by modulating WNT signaling, while midbrain organoids utilize FGF8 to promote the development of dopaminergic neurons (**Figure 5**). These region-specific protocols allow the production of region-specific organoids, such as the hippocampus or cerebellum [9]. Guided protocols often achieve greater cellular diversity and functional specialization compared to unguided methods, making them particularly valuable for studying region-specific neurodevelopmental disorders. Examples include forebrain organoids for investigating autism spectrum disorders [25] and hippocampal organoids for studying epilepsy [26].

Innovations in culture systems have significantly improved the scalability and functionality of brain organoids. Microfluidic platforms and bioreactors enhance reproducibility, while the integration of vascular-like structures via co-culture with endothelial cells or perfusable microfluidic channels addresses challenges such as necrotic core formation [27]. Techniques like engineering molds and 3D printing enable the assembly of organoids from distinct brain regions, forming "assembloids" that model inter-regional connectivity [28, 29] These advanced models have been used to study critical developmental processes, including GABAergic neuron migration from ventral telencephalic progenitors to the cortical plate [10, 30, 31] and the formation of long-range neuronal tracts, including cortico-striatal and cortico-thalamic tracts [16]. Organoids co-cultured with non-neural tissues, such as muscle tissues, have demonstrated the ability of organoid neurons to functionally innervate non-neural tissues, opening new avenues for regenerative medicine research [32, 33].

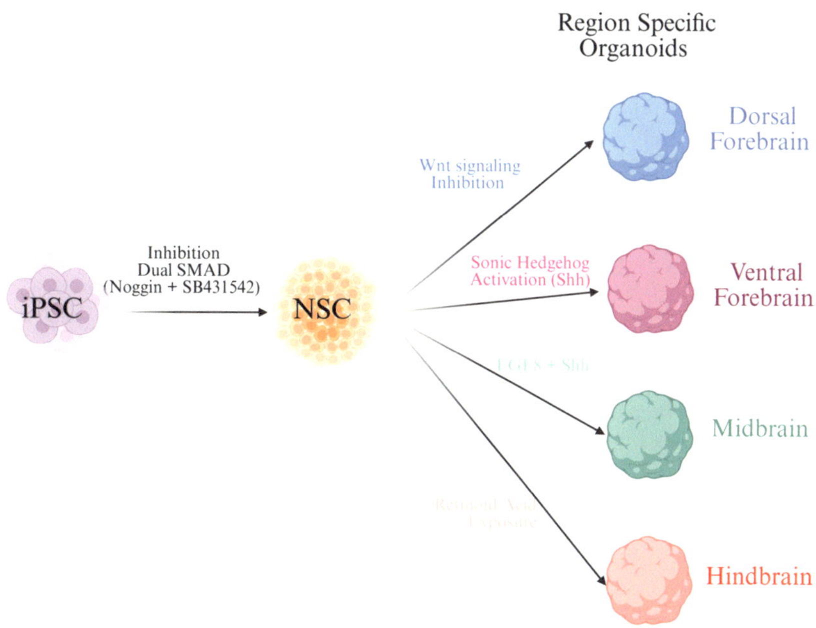

Figure 5.
Guided differentiation of neural stem cells (NSCs) into distinct brain-region-specific organoids. Key signaling pathways, including Wnt inhibition for dorsal forebrain, Sonic Hedgehog (Shh) activation for ventral forebrain, FGF8 + Shh for midbrain, and retinoic acid exposure for hindbrain, direct NSCs toward specialized neural structures, modeling in vivo neurodevelopment. Created with BioRender.com.

Further innovations include delivering localized developmental morphogens to induce multiple brain regions within a single organoid. For instance, introducing a Sonic Hedgehog (SHH) gradient into forebrain organoids facilitates spatial patterning along both dorso-ventral and antero-posterior axes [34]. These advances broaden the applicability of brain organoids for studying complex developmental and disease mechanisms.

4.2 Cellular composition and organization of cortical organoids

Cortical brain organoids exhibit diverse cell populations, including radial glial cells, excitatory and inhibitory neurons, astrocytes, oligodendrocytes, and microglia, reflecting key features of human brain development (**Figure 6**). Single-cell RNA sequencing has further demonstrated that gene expression in cortical brain organoid cells closely mirrors patterns observed in fetal brain tissue, except for the increased activity of genes associated with metabolic stress in radial glial cells and intermediate progenitor cells, specific cell populations, likely due to oxygen limitations at the organoid's core [34].

4.2.1 Neuroepithelial layers

In the initial stages of organoid development (within 5–7 days), neuroepithelial layers form and differentiate into radial glial cells. These cells act as progenitors and scaffolds for neuronal migration, mimicking the ventricular zone (VZ) observed during early brain development.

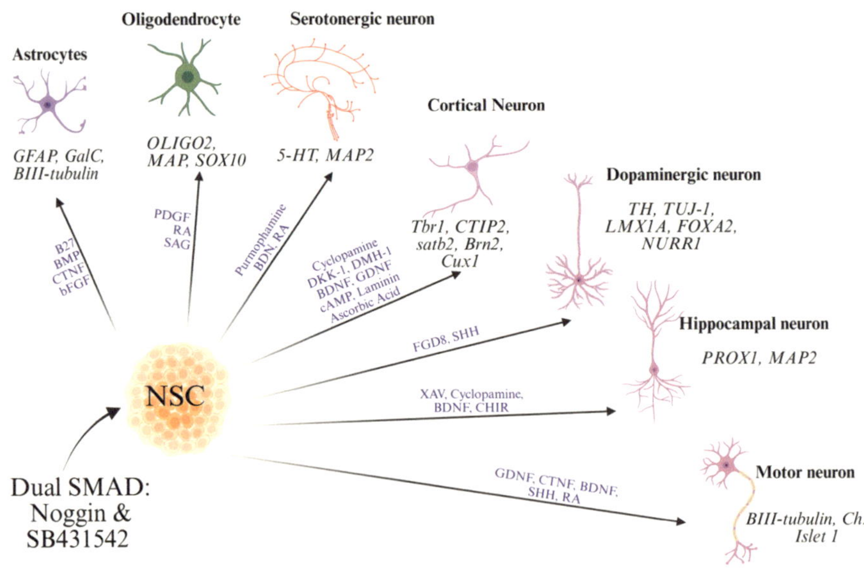

Figure 6.
Differentiation of neural stem cells (NSCs) into various specialized cell types, guided by specific molecular signals. NSCs serve as the progenitor population, differentiating into neurons, astrocytes, oligodendrocytes, microglia, ependymal cells, radial glia, and neural crest cells. Each lineage is regulated by distinct transcription factors and signaling cues, including Neurogenin 2 and NeuroD1 for neuronal differentiation, Notch and NF1 for astrocytes, Olig2 and Sox10 for oligodendrocytes, PU.1 and IRF8 for microglia, FoxJ1 and Notch for ependymal cells, Hes1 and Hes5 for radial glia, and Wnt, BMP, and FGF for neural crest-derived populations. This structured framework provides insight into the molecular mechanisms driving neural fate specification, relevant for both developmental neurobiology and translational applications. Created with BioRender.com.

4.2.2 Cortical-like structures

By 20–30 days, cerebral organoids self-organize into early cortical structures resembling the developing human cortex. These structures include an apical ventricular zone, intermediate zone, and outer cortical plate. Excitatory pyramidal neurons and inhibitory interneurons emerge during this period, modeling early neuronal differentiation and the establishment of basic cortical architecture, comparable to the first trimester of human brain development [12].

4.2.3 Synaptic connectivity and network formation

At 2–3 months, cortical brain organoids demonstrate synaptogenesis, evidenced by the expression of presynaptic proteins (e.g., SYN1, GluNR1) and postsynaptic markers (e.g., PSD95) [35, 36]. While these molecular markers suggest synapse formation, their presence alone does not confirm functional synaptogenesis.

To assess functional maturation, electrophysiological techniques such as whole-cell patch-clamp recordings have been used. Trujillo et al. [37] conducted comprehensive studies using multi-electrode arrays (MEAs) to monitor the neuroelectrical activities of cerebral organoids over a span of 10 months [37]. They observed a progressive increase in firing rates, burst frequency, synchronicity, and population spiking, indicating the development of highly connected neural networks. Notably, after approximately six months in culture, organoids exhibited robust oscillatory activity, which was correlated with the emergence of GABAergic interneurons constituting about 10–15% of the neuronal population. This suggests that GABAergic transmission is essential for the maintenance of oscillatory activity [38, 39].

Further insights were provided by Fair et al. [39], who utilized MEAs to detect spontaneous electrical activity in brain organoids from day 34 onwards. They reported a progressive increase in electrophysiological properties, including synchronized burst firing and elevated mean firing rates compared to 2D monolayer neurons, highlighting the enhanced network complexity in organoids [39, 40]. Complementary to electrophysiological recordings, calcium imaging studies have visualized spontaneous calcium transients and synchronized activity across neuronal populations within organoids, providing further evidence of functional synaptic networks [41]. Collectively, these experimental approaches confirm that brain organoids not only form synaptic structures but also develop functional neural networks, making them valuable models for studying human brain development and neurological disorders.

4.2.4 Incorporation of glial cells

Glial cell populations enhance the physiological relevance of cortical organoids. Astrocytes typically emerge after 2–3 months of culture and increase with time in culture [12], contributing to synaptogenesis, synapse maintenance, and metabolic support [42]. By 6 months, they can constitute up to 50% of cells, identified by GFAP and S100P expression [22]. Oligodendrocytes appear in cultures extending beyond 4–6 months, enabling myelination in mature organoids [43]. Microglia, essential for immune functions and synaptic pruning [44], are less consistently incorporated and often require exogenous methods for reliable inclusion, reflecting technical challenges in replicating the complete brain microenvironment [45].

4.3 Organoids as models for human-specific aspects of brain development

Now that we have explored the cellular composition and organization of cortical organoids, let us delve deeper into what makes these systems uniquely suited for studying human-specific aspects of brain development. Organoids provide an unprecedented window into processes that are not easily replicated in animal models, such as the complexity of radial glial scaffolds, the intricacies of neuronal migration and cortical folding, and the distinct transcriptomic patterns that define human neurodevelopment.

4.3.1 Radial glial scaffold formation

One of the first human-specific traits that organoids recapitulate is the remarkable complexity of radial glial cells. In the human brain, these cells exhibit prolonged neurogenic potential and intricate organization, forming scaffolds that guide migrating neurons and facilitate cortical expansion. Organoids recapitulate these human-specific traits, offering insights into the evolutionary divergence of cortical development. For example, Nowakowski et al. [46] used organoids to reveal how radial glial fibers support neuronal migration and cortical folding, features that set human neurodevelopment apart from other species [46]. These findings extend beyond basic science; they have illuminated the pathology of Fukuyama muscular dystrophy, where disruptions in radial glial fiber migration impair cortical architecture and neuronal positioning [47].

4.3.2 Neuronal migration and cortical folding

As organoids mature, they unveil the dynamic choreography of neuronal migration, where neurons glide along radial glial fibers to reach their destined cortical layers [48]. As organoids mature, they unveil the dynamic choreography of neuronal migration, where neurons glide along radial glial fibers to reach their destined cortical layers. These studies have also identified molecules such as HAPLN1, lumican, and collagen I as key drivers of this cortical folding, while the degradation of hyaluronic acid (HA) disrupts these folds. Such insights make organoids indispensable for unraveling the etiology of cortical malformations, such as lissencephaly how disruptions in ECM-mediated folding can reveal the underlying mechanisms of these disorders, advancing our understanding of neurodevelopmental abnormalities [49].

4.3.3 Disease modeling

Beyond structural insights, organoids have transformed our ability to model neurodevelopmental diseases. Consider the case of Zika virus, where organoids revealed how the virus selectively targets neural progenitor cells, leading to microcephaly [50]. Similarly, mutations associated with autism spectrum disorder (ASD), such as CHD8, have been studied using forebrain organoids, exposing disruptions in neuronal differentiation and synapse formation [25]. These discoveries are not just academic; they pave the way for potential therapeutic interventions, offering hope for conditions previously shrouded in mystery. Later in this chapter, we will explore these disease models in greater depth to uncover the full potential of organoids as tools for understanding and addressing neurodevelopmental disorders.

4.3.4 Human-specific transcriptomics

Having explored how organoids recapitulate key cellular and structural aspects of the developing brain, we now turn to another critical dimension: their ability to capture human-specific transcriptional landscapes. Comparative transcriptomic analyses between organoids and primary human brain tissues have shown that organoids faithfully model the gene expression profiles of human brain tissues, particularly during early developmental stages [51]. In a landmark study, Uzquiano et al. [34] constructed a comprehensive "tree of life" depicting cellular differentiation within organoids. This map revealed the stepwise progression of stem cells into radial glial cells, neurons, and eventually specialized subtypes, reflecting the developmental trajectories of the human brain [34]. By comparing this tree to its mouse counterpart, the study revealed unique human gene expression patterns and transcription factors, highlighting the evolutionary divergence in cortical development.

Notably, Uzquiano and co-workers have also explored early developmental processes typically confined to the womb, observing the early stages diversification of callosal projection neurons, cells critical for interhemispheric communication [34]. These neurons, more abundant and diverse in humans than other species, are thought to contribute to the expansion of the human cortex. The observed patterns in organoids not only validate their relevance as models of human neurodevelopment but also highlight their potential to address evolutionary questions.

By bridging the gap between in vitro models and in vivo human development, transcriptomic studies of brain organoids are redefining our understanding of human neurobiology. They offer not only a window into the molecular mechanisms driving brain development but also a platform for investigating how deviations from these processes contribute to disease. As we advance, integrating transcriptomic insights with other omics approaches will undoubtedly expand the scope of organoids, enabling even deeper exploration of human-specific brain features and shaping the future of neuroscience research.

5. Applications of organoid technology in brain development and disease research

5.1 Understanding healthy brain development versus disease states

Brain organoids have revolutionized our ability to study healthy brain development and its pathological deviations. Previously, we discussed how these models replicate the three-dimensional architecture, cellular diversity, and spatiotemporal gene expression patterns of the developing human brain. These features enable the exploration of key developmental processes, including neurogenesis, radial glial cell expansion, neuronal differentiation, and synaptic network formation. Building on this foundation, this section highlights examples of how brain organoids have been applied to uncover insights into both normal brain development and the disruptions caused by various disease states.

5.1.1 Insights into nonpathogenic brain development

Brain organoids provide a unique platform for studying sex-specific differences in brain development, revealing distinctions in gene expression and hormonal signaling.

Male-derived brain organoids show elevated androgen receptor activity, which influences neuronal differentiation and network formation, while female-derived organoids display estrogen receptor signaling patterns that impact synaptic density and maturation [52]. These findings have profound implications for understanding sex-related variability in neurodevelopmental disorders, such as autism spectrum disorder (ASD) and attention-deficit/hyperactivity disorder (ADHD), which differ in prevalence and clinical presentation between sexes. Future research integrating organoid data with clinical findings aims to address how these differences contribute to disease susceptibility and guide the development of sex-specific therapeutic approaches.

5.1.2 Modeling neurodevelopmental disorders

Cerebral organoids can facilitate understanding neurodevelopmental diseases, including microcephaly-related disease (e.g., autosomal recessive primary microcephaly, MCPH), ASD, Rett's syndrome (RTT), Timothy's syndrome (TS), and Down's syndrome (DS), Leigh's syndrome (LS).

MCPH is a neurodevelopmental disease in which head circumference is markedly reduced, directly characterized by a smaller cerebral cortex [53]. To model MCPH, iPSCs-derived cerebral organoids with mutations in genes KNL1 and NARS1 displayed a reduction in neural progenitors and a defect in the formation of neural rosette structure, mirroring the cortical underdevelopment observed in patients [54]. Similarly, cerebral organoids have also been applied to understand pathogen-caused microcephaly. Using human forebrain organoids, it was found that ZIKA virus-encoded protein NS2A reduced radial glial cell proliferation by causing deficits in adherens junctions and scaffolding of radial glial fibers [55]. Together, these studies demonstrate that deep insights into MCPH, caused by either genetic mutations or pathogen infections, can be readily gained through the lens of human brain organoids.

In ASD, which are characterized by impaired social communication, patient-derived organoids reveal altered neurogenesis and cortical lamination, with specific mutations, such as overexpression of Forkhead Box protein G1 (FOXG1), contributing to these phenotypes [56].

Organoids from ASD patients have shown disrupted cortical lamination among other phenotypes [57]. A recent study by directly inducing ASD iPSCs into neurons and forebrain organoids revealed a temporal dysregulation of specific gene networks that caused marked abnormalities of cortical neuron development [58]. Organoid models have also highlighted shifts in GABAergic lineage determination, which are consistently observed across different ASD systems [59]. These findings underscore the potential of organoids to elucidate disease-specific mechanisms and identify therapeutic targets.

In the past, research on RTT primarily relied on post-mortem human brain samples [60] and transgenic mouse models [61] . However, these approaches faced limitations, such as scarce human tissue availability and incomplete replication of RTT phenotypes in animal models. RTT, caused by pathogenic variants in the MECP2 gene, has been further elucidated using patient iPSC-derived cerebral organoids. These organoids demonstrated how MECP2 deficiency disrupts neural progenitor function and neuronal migration by regulating microRNAs, including miR-199 and miR-214 [62]. Such findings not only clarify the cellular mechanisms underlying RTT but also highlight the potential of organoids in overcoming the limitations of traditional models.

TS, a rare neurodevelopmental disorder caused by pathogenic variants in the CACNA1C gene encoding the L-type voltage-gated calcium channel (CaV1.2), has been extensively studied using cerebral organoids. These models reveal that gain-of-function variants in CaV1.2 lead to prolonged channel opening, excessive calcium influx, and dysregulated calcium signaling, which disrupt neuronal differentiation, excitability, and synaptic connectivity [63]. Advanced techniques like calcium fluorescence imaging and patch-clamp recordings have shown abnormal oscillatory calcium activity and impaired network synchronization in TS organoids, mirroring patient phenotypes. Additionally, organoids have facilitated preclinical testing of a selective antisense oligonucleotides (ASOs) therapeutic approach for TS [26]. These findings underscore the utility of organoids in uncovering disease mechanisms and testing targeted therapies for TS.

DS is a complex genetic disorder primarily caused by trisomy 21, the presence of an extra copy of chromosome 21, though mosaicism and partial trisomy can also contribute to the condition. It is characterized by intellectual disability, a reduced brain size, and altered neurogenesis. Notable structural changes in the DS brain include a smaller cerebellum, reduced cerebral hemispheres, and an imbalance in excitatory and inhibitory neurons.

iPSC-derived forebrain organoids from DS patients have revealed an overproduction of OLIG2+ progenitors, resulting in an excess of inhibitory interneurons (GABAergic neurons). This finding aligns with the disrupted excitatory-inhibitory balance observed in DS patients [64]. Similarly, brain organoids have been employed to study LS, a rare inherited neurometabolic disorder linked to defects in the mitochondrial respiratory chain. LS patient-derived cerebral organoids exhibit impaired neural epithelial bud generation, reduced size, and abnormal cortical architecture by 100 days, highlighting their potential for phenotypic characterization and mechanistic insights into this disorder [65].

5.1.3 Neurodegenerative disorders

Brain organoids serve as a valuable model system for investigating the mechanisms underlying neurodegenerative disorders, including Alzheimer's and Parkinson's disease. Alzheimer's disease is the most common neurodegenerative disease, which can be studied by using organoid models that capture pathologies and allow disease mechanisms to be investigated. Multiple groups have shown that iPSC-organoids harboring familial AD (FAD) mutations also develop Aβ pathology, providing important evidence that endogenous expression levels of AD-associated mutations can drive pathology in vitro, avoiding potential artifacts associated with overexpression [66]. In the context of (PD), recent advancements have been made in the development of Midbrain organoids (MBOs) models derived from hiPSCs that consider key pathophysiological mechanisms such as alpha-synuclein (α-Syn), lewy bodies, dopamine loss, and microglia activation [67].

The potential of brain organoids extends into modeling age-related and neurodegenerative diseases, as well as genetic disorders. Organoids have been utilized to study Alzheimer's disease (AD), Parkinson's disease (PD), and Huntington's disease (HD). For example, organoids derived from familial Alzheimer's patients exhibit hallmark amyloid-beta plaques and tau tangles, which are critical features of AD pathology. The development of amyloid plaques in these organoids occurs as early as day 30 of differentiation, and by day 60, tau hyperphosphorylation is observed, mimicking the temporal progression of the disease in vivo. These organoids also demonstrate aberrant synaptic activity and neural network dysfunction, which can be used for therapeutic screening and testing drug efficacy [68]. The ability to model these features in vitro has enabled researchers to evaluate potential treatments targeting amyloid-beta accumulation and tau pathology in a more human-relevant system than animal models, which often fail to fully replicate human AD characteristics.

5.2 Organoids for personalized medicine

As discussed in the previous section, the combination of the hiPSC technology with the cortical brain organoid platform has allowed modeling of both human brain development and brain disorders [69]. Hence, cortical brain organoids have emerged as a powerful tool in personalized medicine, enabling the replication of individual patient conditions and the customization of therapeutic approaches. A significant challenge in studying brain development and neurological diseases is the limited access to live human brain tissue. By utilizing patient-derived iPSCs, cortical brain organoids can recapitulate complex neurological disease phenotypes, providing a personalized system for studying disease mechanisms and testing therapeutic strategies [10]. This approach would facilitate drug screening before initiating treatment, offering a promising platform for conducting "clinical trials in a dish." For example, organoids have been generated from glioblastoma patients' tumor cells and used to screen cancer drugs to determine the most promising options before initiating treatment [69]. iPSCs derived neurons from a Timothy syndrome patient's iPSCs exhibited corresponding neuronal hyperexcitability that was rescued by roscovitine, validating a potential therapy [69]. Cortical brain organoids could eventually enable routine testing of therapies on patient-derived models to determine optimal personalized approaches. Though still early, organoids present opportunities to tailor medicine and improve clinical outcomes that are unprecedented with traditional methods. Challenges remain in time to the availability of models for individual patient decisions, adult-like maturation, and validation of organoid-based assays, but precision medicine approaches are clearly on the horizon [70].

5.3 Potential applications in regenerative medicine

The promise of cortical brain organoids extends to regenerative medicine, where they could aid in repairing or replacing damaged brain tissue. Advances in bioengineering, such as incorporating vascular-like structures, improve the viability of transplantable organoid grafts. For example, preclinical studies have shown that cortical brain organoids transplanted into rodent brains integrate with host vasculature and form functional synaptic connections, suggesting potential applications in treating traumatic brain injuries or neurodegenerative conditions [27, 71].

In addition to organoid-based approaches, recent advances in cell therapy and direct reprogramming offer complementary strategies to restore neural function in degenerative conditions. For instance, transplanting healthy dopaminergic neurons into the brains of PD patients aims to restore dopaminergic activity lost due to the degeneration of substantia nigra neurons. The transplanted neurons are typically derived from hiPSCs and are differentiated into midbrain dopaminergic neurons before transplantation. These cells are then stereotaxically implanted into the striatum, where they can integrate into the host neural circuitry. Then, the transplanted dopaminergic neurons establish synaptic connections with host neurons, restoring dopaminergic signaling pathways [72]. These neurons survive, mature, and improve motor function in animal models of PD. Ongoing clinical trials assess the safety and efficacy of this method in human patients [73].

In parallel, direct reprogramming offers an alternative regenerative strategy by converting resident glial cells, such as astrocytes, into functional neurons within the adult brain. This approach leverages the plasticity of astrocytes and their abundance in the central nervous system [74]. One of the key mechanisms involves the knockdown of polypyrimidine tract-binding protein 1 (PTBP1), a regulator of RNA splicing that suppresses neuronal gene expression in non-neuronal cells. By reducing PTBP1 levels, astrocytes can be reprogrammed into neurons without passing through a pluripotent intermediate state. This has been achieved using adeno-associated virus (AAV) vectors delivering short hairpin RNA (shRNA) targeting PTBP1 under the control of the glial fibrillary acidic protein (GFAP) promoter, ensuring specificity to astrocytes. In mouse models of neurodegenerative diseases, such as PD, this strategy has led to the generation of functional neurons that integrate into existing neural circuits and ameliorate disease symptoms [75]. Additionally, antisense oligonucleotides (ASOs) targeting PTBP1 mRNA have been employed to achieve similar reprogramming effects. ASOs offer advantages in terms of dosage control and reduced risk of insertional mutagenesis compared to viral vectors. The use of ASOs has demonstrated the successful conversion of astrocytes into dopaminergic neurons in vivo, leading to functional recovery in PD mouse models [76].

These regenerative approaches, organoid transplantation and direct reprogramming, offer complementary strategies to replenish lost neurons and restore neural function. Ongoing research aims to enhance reprogramming efficiency, ensure the safety of newly generated neurons, and address challenges such as immune rejection. Furthermore, to enhance organoid functionality and tailor them for patient-specific therapies, many research groups are exploring engineering approaches using biocompatible scaffolds and CRISPR-Cas9 gene editing. Ethical considerations, such as defining criteria for neural consciousness and addressing graft-host compatibility, remain crucial to advancing these therapies responsibly.

By integrating organoid transplantation, direct reprogramming, and advanced bioengineering, regenerative medicine is poised to transform treatments for neurodegenerative diseases and brain injuries. These advancements bridge the gap between basic research and clinical application, driving progress toward innovative, personalized therapeutic solutions.

6. Challenges and limitations of organoid models

While cortical brain organoids are valuable models for studying human brain development and disease, they are not perfect replicas of the human prefrontal cortex. These models effectively capture key aspects of brain structure, cellular composition, and neural activity, yet they fall short in replicating certain critical features. For instance, cortical brain organoids often lack specific cell types, such as vascular endothelial cells and microglia [77] which are essential for modeling neurovascular and neuroimmune interactions [78]. One of the most significant limitations is the absence of vascularization, which constrains their size and complexity. Without a functional blood supply, the diffusion of nutrients and oxygen is inefficient, resulting in hypoxia, cellular stress, and necrosis in the organoid core [79].

Despite their promise, cortical brain organoids also raise important ethical considerations. These include concerns about cell sourcing, donor consent, commercialization, and their use in animal or human studies. As human brain organoids become more advanced, discussions surrounding their potential for consciousness, while speculative at present, underscore the need for proactive ethical and legal frameworks [80]. For example, consent issues unique to brain organoid research, such as the potential for transplantation and use in invasive studies, require careful consideration. Similarly, the transplantation of organoids into animals presents challenges related to animal welfare and the need for stricter evaluation of research purposes and impacts [80]. Although the current generation of organoids is far from achieving consciousness, rapid advancements in the field highlight the importance of clear guidelines to prevent misuse and maintain public trust. Ethical and regulatory efforts must keep pace with innovation to support responsible development while addressing societal concerns [81].

7. Future directions: The next frontier in brain development research

7.1 Advancing brain organoids with microfluidics and brain-on-a-chip platforms

As organoid technology continues to evolve, the future holds promise for more sophisticated models that closely replicate human brain function. Traditional single-region organoids have provided valuable insights into early brain development and disease; however, their inability to fully mimic the complexity of the human brain, including functional integration and physiological interactions, is a limitation that the increasing generation of assembloids aims to address. One emerging direction is the development of brain-on-a-chip platforms, which combine organoid technology with microfluidic systems to create dynamic and physiologically relevant environments such as brain blood barrier (BBB). Recent innovations, such as microfluidic devices for controlled nutrient diffusion and waste removal, have supported the extended maturation and enhanced functionality of cerebral organoids [82].

By combining organoid cultures with these advanced technologies, it is possible to better capture the neurovascular interactions, metabolic conditions, and other physiologically relevant features absent in traditional models. These advancements position brain-on-a-chip platforms as indispensable tools for drug screening, disease modeling, and understanding complex brain disorders with unprecedented precision.

7.2 Multiorgan systems: Expanding the scope of organotypic research

Another promising frontier is the integration of brain organoids with other organoid models to create multiorgan systems that simulate systemic interactions within the human body. For example, linking brain organoids with vascular, liver, or gut organoids could enable to better simulate the interactions between the brain and peripheral organs, such as studying cancer metastasis [83]. This approach is particularly valuable for exploring diseases such as Alzheimer's and Parkinson's, where systemic inflammation and peripheral organ dysfunction are critical contributors.

Multiorgan systems also open avenues for modeling complex drug interactions and studying the impact of metabolic disorders on neurodevelopment and aging. Despite challenges, including synchronizing the maturation and functional integration of multiple organoids, advances in microfluidics, bioprinting, and organ-on-a-chip technologies are rapidly overcoming these hurdles. These integrated systems promise to revolutionize our understanding of the brain's interactions with the body, providing comprehensive models for systemic diseases and therapeutic testing.

7.3 Extending applications to peripheral nerve regeneration

Building on the multiorgan systems discussion, peripheral nerve regeneration represents a promising frontier for organoid and co-culture technologies. While CNS modeling has been the primary focus, peripheral nerve regeneration (PNS) offers unique opportunities to address challenges in neural repair. Koyanagi et al. [84] developed a dorsal root ganglion (DRG)-derived organotypic model using rat DRG explants cultured in a 3D organoid system [84]. These cultures retained key PNS features, including sensory neuron identity and organized neurite outgrowth, serving as a platform for studying axonal growth and targeted connectivity. Similarly, co-culture systems incorporating DRG organoids derived from human pluripotent stem cells express sensory neuron markers (TrkA, TrkB, and TrkC) and establish functional connections with cortical organoids, as demonstrated by Kim et al. [85] using rabies virus tracing and calcium imaging [85].

The PNS microenvironment plays a critical role in peripheral regeneration. A 2022 study showed that 3D scaffolds combining DRG neurons, Schwann cells, and endothelial cells significantly enhanced axonal growth and neurotrophic factor release (NGF, VEGF) via PI3K-Akt and MAPK pathways [86]. Additionally, Pereira et al. [87] created sensorimotor organoids containing both motor and sensory neurons, validating functional neuromuscular junctions and sensory–motor interactions, highlighting the potential for PNS–CNS integration [87].

Expanding organoid-based models for peripheral nerve regeneration is essential for bridging CNS and PNS research. Innovations in bioprinting and synthetic scaffolds address challenges such as extracellular matrix replication and culture stability, paving the way for unified, translational neural repair systems. These advancements promise to deepen our understanding of neural repair dynamics, offering comprehensive tools for CNS and PNS integration.

7.4 Leveraging advanced imaging, genetic editing, and machine learning

To further enhance the utility of brain organoids, it is necessary to integrate them with cutting-edge technologies such as advanced imaging, gene editing, and machine learning. Advanced imaging modalities, such as two-photon microscopy and live-cell imaging, enable real-time tracking of organoid development, neural network formation, and synaptic activity at high resolution. These technologies provide detailed mapping of brain structure and function, offering insights into normal development and disease mechanisms.

Genetic manipulation, particularly CRISPR-Cas9 editing, is another transformative tool. By introducing or modifying specific genes within organoids, it becomes possible to model genetic disorders and investigate the effects of mutations on neurodevelopment. For instance, recent studies using CRISPR in brain organoids have identified critical genes involved in microcephaly [88], and similar approaches are being used to model autism spectrum disorder (ASD) by introducing specific mutations in candidate genes such as CHD8 [89].

Machine learning (ML) is invaluable for analyzing the vast datasets generated by organoid experiments. ML algorithms can process imaging data, predict cellular behaviors, and uncover patterns in gene expression linked to disease phenotypes.

This approach accelerates the identification of biomarkers and therapeutic targets, streamlining drug discovery and disease modeling.

7.5 Exploring organoid intelligence: A paradigm shift in Biocomputing

An exciting and transformative frontier is the concept of Organoid Intelligence (OI), where brain organoids function as living biocomputational systems. By leveraging the inherent properties of neural tissue, such as synaptic plasticity, network formation, and adaptive learning, OI systems blur the line between biological cognition and artificial intelligence [90].

This biocomputational paradigm integrates cerebral organoids with advanced electrophysiological and optical systems to establish a two-way interface for neural activity monitoring and stimulation. Multielectrode arrays (MEAs) and optogenetics enable precise stimulation and recording of neural activity, translating the organoid's biological signals into machine-readable inputs. Computational systems process this data to adaptively stimulate the organoid, fostering feedback loops essential for learning. For example, in a pioneering application, researchers trained an organoid to play "Pong," where it received sensory inputs as electrical signals and responded with motor-like outputs, refining its performance over time through trial and error [91].

OI systems also integrate machine learning algorithms to decode the organoid's neural dynamics. Techniques like deep learning and network analysis extract meaningful patterns from the complex and nonlinear neural activity, allowing researchers to understand and optimize the system's cognitive processes. Concurrently, bioengineering innovations, such as microfluidic platforms and chemical signal modulators, enhance the organoid's computational capacity by providing fine-tuned control over its microenvironment.

The implications of OI extend far beyond technical curiosity. These systems provide unparalleled opportunities to study the biological basis of learning and memory, develop neuromorphic hardware inspired by biological principles, and even explore the ethical dimensions of creating intelligence in vitro. OI bridges the gap between synthetic intelligence and natural cognition, establishing a novel platform for both discovery and application. As OI evolves, it shifts organoid research from a focus on understanding development and disease to exploring intelligence itself, offering a glimpse into the future of biocomputing and cognition studies.

7.6 Ethical and regulatory framework

As brain organoid technology progresses rapidly, addressing the ethical and regulatory challenges becomes indispensable to guide responsible research and translation. The ethical discourse surrounding organoids spans several critical areas, including cell source provenance, xenotransplantation risks, commercialization, and emerging concerns about potential consciousness or sentience [92].

7.6.1 Cell source and consent

Most brain organoids are derived from human pluripotent stem cells (PSCs), including embryonic stem cells (ESCs) and induced pluripotent stem cells (iPSCs). Ethical concerns arise regarding informed consent, donor privacy, and the moral status of ESCs. iPSCs partially mitigate some concerns by using reprogrammed adult cells, but questions about consent for future uses and donor anonymity remain [93].

Moreover, the potential for generating organoids with increasingly complex structures raises debates about the moral considerations tied to human tissue complexity [94].

7.6.2 Xenotransplantation and animal models

Transplanting human brain organoids into animal brains (xenotransplantation) is a powerful approach to study integration and maturation in vivo. However, it raises ethical issues related to chimerism, species boundaries, and animal welfare. Regulatory frameworks are still evolving to address these concerns, balancing scientific benefit against moral implications of creating human-animal neural chimeras [95].

7.6.3 Commercialization and intellectual property

The rapid development of organoid technologies has generated commercial interest, prompting concerns over equitable access, the patenting of biological materials, and potential exploitation. There is a need for transparent policies to regulate commercialization pathways while safeguarding public interests and promoting open scientific collaboration [92].

7.6.4 Consciousness and sentience

One of the most debated topics is whether advanced brain organoids could develop forms of consciousness or sentience. Although current organoids lack vascularization and full structural complexity, ongoing advances prompt preemptive ethical reflections on potential sentient states and corresponding research oversight [96, 97]. The concept of "moral status" for organoids remains speculative but emphasizes the need for continuous ethical evaluation as technology evolves.

7.6.5 Regulatory landscape

Regulatory bodies, including the International Society for Stem Cell Research (ISSCR), have issued guidelines encouraging rigorous oversight of organoid research, recommending transparency, ethical review, and public engagement [98]. National regulations vary, and harmonization remains a challenge, underscoring the importance of global discourse to foster responsible innovation.

In summary, the ethical and regulatory framework for brain organoids must evolve alongside scientific advances. Proactive policies and interdisciplinary dialog involving scientists, ethicists, policymakers, and the public are essential to navigate these challenges, ensuring that organoid research progresses ethically, responsibly, and with societal trust.

8. Concluding remarks

The advances in brain organoid research, combined with innovations in microphysiological systems and cutting-edge techniques, have revolutionized our understanding of brain development and disorders. From elucidating developmental processes to modeling complex diseases, brain organoids provide an unprecedented platform for translational research. By incorporating technologies such as microfluidics, genetic editing, and machine learning, these models are not only refining our understanding of the brain but also transforming drug discovery and therapeutic development.

While challenges remain, such as enhancing organoid maturity, functional integration, and scalability, ongoing innovations in biomimetic engineering, multiorgan systems, and bioinformatics promise to address these limitations. The emergence of platforms like organoid intelligence also paves the way for groundbreaking studies in cognition and biocomputing.

Ultimately, the integration of brain organoid technology with other advanced systems underscores a shift toward more comprehensive, physiologically relevant models. These advancements hold the potential to bridge critical gaps in neuroscience, offering transformative opportunities for understanding, diagnosing, and treating neurological and systemic diseases. As the field evolves, ethical considerations and standardization will be key to ensuring the responsible application of this promising technology.

Conflict of interest

The authors declare no conflict of interest.

Author details

Farjana Yasmin, Rodrigo Cristofoletti and Janny Piñeiro-Llanes*
Department of Pharmaceutics, University of Florida, Orlando, Florida, USA

*Address all correspondence to: jpineiro@ufl.edu

References

[1] Huch M, Koo BK. Modeling mouse and human development using organoid cultures. Development (Cambridge). 2015;**142**:3113-3125

[2] Iefremova V, Manikakis G, Krefft O, et al. An organoid-based model of cortical development identifies non-cell-autonomous defects in Wnt signaling contributing to Miller-Dieker syndrome. Cell Reports. 2017;**19**:50-59

[3] Corrò C, Novellasdemunt L, Li VSW. A brief history of organoids. American Journal of Physiology-Cell Physiology. 2020;**319**:151-165

[4] Lee C, Bendriem RM, Wu WW, et al. 3D brain organoids derived from pluripotent stem cells: Promising experimental models for brain development and neurodegenerative disorders. Journal of Biomedical Science. 2017;**24**:59

[5] The Society for Neuroscience. In: Brain Facts, a Primer on the Brain and Nervous System. 8th ed. Washington (DC): Society for Neuroscience; 2018

[6] Watson C, Kirkcaldie M, Paxinos G. The human cerebral cortex. In: Watson C, Kirkcaldie M, Paxinos G, editors. The Brain. San Diego: Academic Press; 2010. pp. 97-108

[7] Konrad K, Firk C, Uhlhaas PJ. Brain development during. Adolescence. 2013;**110**:425-432

[8] Lancaster MA, Renner M, Martin C-A, et al. Cerebral organoids model human brain development and microcephaly. Nature. 2013;**501**:373-379

[9] Paşca AM, Sloan SA, Clarke LE, et al. Functional cortical neurons and astrocytes from human pluripotent stem cells in 3D culture. Nature Methods. 2015;**12**:671-678

[10] Birey F, Andersen J, Makinson CD, et al. Assembly of functionally integrated human forebrain spheroids. Nature. 2017;**545**:54-59

[11] 'Mini Brains' are not like the real thing | Scientific American. Available from: https://www.scientificamerican.com/article/mini-brains-are-not-like-the-real-thing/ [Accessed: April 4, 2025]

[12] Quadrato G, Nguyen T, Macosko EZ, et al. Cell diversity and network dynamics in photosensitive human brain organoids. Nature. 2017;**545**:48-53

[13] Miura Y, Li M-Y, Birey F, et al. Generation of human striatal organoids and cortico-striatal assembloids from human pluripotent stem cells. Nature Biotechnology. 2020;**38**:1421-1430

[14] Sakaguchi H, Kadoshima T, Soen M, et al. Generation of functional hippocampal neurons from self-organizing human embryonic stem cell-derived dorsomedial telencephalic tissue. Nature Communications. 2015;**6**:8896

[15] Ozone C, Suga H, Eiraku M, et al. Functional anterior pituitary generated in self-organizing culture of human embryonic stem cells. Nature Communications. 2016;7:10351

[16] Xiang Y, Tanaka Y, Cakir B, et al. hESC-derived thalamic organoids form reciprocal projections when fused with cortical organoids. Cell Stem Cell. 2019;**24**:487-497.e7

[17] Jo J, Xiao Y, Sun AX, et al. Midbrain-like organoids from human

pluripotent stem cells contain functional dopaminergic and neuromelanin-producing neurons. Cell Stem Cell. 2016;**19**:248-257

[18] Muguruma K, Nishiyama A, Kawakami H, et al. Self-organization of polarized cerebellar tissue in 3D culture of human pluripotent stem cells. Cell Reports. 2015;**10**:537-550

[19] Strang KH, Golde TE, Giasson BI. MAPT mutations, tauopathy, and mechanisms of neurodegeneration. Laboratory Investigation. 2019;**99**:912-928

[20] Spillantini MG, Crowther RA, Jakes R, et al. Alpha-synuclein in filamentous inclusions of Lewy bodies from Parkinson's disease and dementia with Lewy bodies. Proceedings of the National Academy of Sciences of the United States of America. 1998;**95**:6469-6473

[21] Seo J, Kritskiy O, Ashley Watson L, et al. Inhibition of p25/Cdk5 attenuates tauopathy in mouse and iPSC models of frontotemporal dementia. The Journal of Neuroscience. 2017;**37**:9917-9924

[22] Velasco S, Kedaigle AJ, Simmons SK, et al. Individual brain organoids reproducibly form cell diversity of the human cerebral cortex. Nature. 2019;**570**:523-527

[23] Theka I, Caiazzo M, Dvoretskova E, et al. Rapid generation of functional dopaminergic neurons from human induced pluripotent stem cells through a single-step procedure using cell lineage transcription factors. Stem Cells Translational Medicine. 2013;**2**:473-479

[24] Bhaduri A, Andrews MG, Mancia Leon W, et al. Cell stress in cortical organoids impairs molecular subtype specification. Nature. 2020;**578**:142-148

[25] Paulsen B, Velasco S, Kedaigle AJ, et al. Autism genes converge on asynchronous development of shared neuron classes. Nature. 2022;**602**:268-273

[26] Chen X, Birey F, Li M-Y, et al. Antisense oligonucleotide therapeutic approach for Timothy syndrome. Nature. 2024;**628**:818-825

[27] Mansour AA, Gonçalves JT, Bloyd CW, et al. An in vivo model of functional and vascularized human brain organoids. Nature Biotechnology. 2018;**36**:432-441

[28] Cassel de Camps C, Rostami S, Xu V, et al. Microfabricated dynamic brain organoid cocultures to assess the effects of surface geometry on assembloid formation. Biotechnology Journal. 2024;**19**:2400070

[29] Roth JG, Brunel LG, Huang MS, et al. Spatially controlled construction of assembloids using bioprinting. Nature Communications. 2023;**14**:4346

[30] Xiang Y, Tanaka Y, Patterson B, et al. Fusion of regionally specified hPSC-derived organoids models human brain development and interneuron migration. Cell Stem Cell. 2017;**21**:383-398.e7

[31] Bagley JA, Reumann D, Bian S, et al. Fused cerebral organoids model interactions between brain regions. Nature Methods. 2017;**14**:743-751

[32] Andersen J, Revah O, Miura Y, et al. Generation of functional human 3D cortico-motor assembloids. Cell. 2020;**183**:1913-1929.e26

[33] Giandomenico SL, Mierau SB, Gibbons GM, et al. Cerebral organoids at the air–liquid interface generate diverse nerve tracts with functional output. Nature Neuroscience. 2019;**22**:669-679

[34] Uzquiano A, Kedaigle AJ, Pigoni M, et al. Proper acquisition of cell class identity in organoids allows definition of fate specification programs of the human cerebral cortex. Cell. 2022;**185**:3770-3788.e27

[35] Yakoub AM. Cerebral organoids exhibit mature neurons and astrocytes and recapitulate electrophysiological activity of the human brain. Neural Regeneration Research. 2019;**14**:757-761

[36] Zafeiriou MP, Bao G, Hudson J, et al. Developmental GABA polarity switch and neuronal plasticity in bioengineered neuronal organoids. Nature Communications. 2020;**11**:1-12

[37] Trujillo CA, Gao R, Negraes PD, et al. Complex oscillatory waves emerging from cortical organoids model early human brain network development. Cell Stem Cell. 2019;**25**:558-569.e7

[38] Zourray C, Kurian MA, Barral S, et al. Electrophysiological properties of human cortical organoids: Current state of the art and future directions. Frontiers in Molecular Neuroscience. 2022;**15**:839366

[39] Fair SR, Julian D, Hartlaub AM, et al. Electrophysiological maturation of cerebral organoids correlates with dynamic morphological and cellular development. Stem Cell Reports. 2020;**15**:855

[40] Tasnim K, Liu J. Emerging bioelectronics for brain organoid electrophysiology. Journal of Molecular Biology. 2021;**434**:167165

[41] Sakaguchi H, Ozaki Y, Ashida T, et al. Self-organized synchronous calcium transients in a cultured human neural network derived from cerebral organoids. Stem Cell Reports. 2019;**13**:458

[42] Sloan SA, Darmanis S, Huber N, et al. Human astrocyte maturation captured in 3D cerebral cortical spheroids derived from pluripotent stem cells. Neuron. 2017;**95**:779-790.e6

[43] Madhavan M, Nevin ZS, Shick HE, et al. Induction of myelinating oligodendrocytes in human cortical spheroids. Nature Methods. 2018;**15**:700-706

[44] Abud EM, Ramirez RN, Martinez ES, et al. iPSC-derived human microglia-like cells to study neurological diseases. Neuron. 2017;**94**:278-293.e9

[45] Ormel PR, Vieira de Sá R, van Bodegraven EJ, et al. Microglia innately develop within cerebral organoids. Nature Communications. 2018;**9**:4167

[46] Nowakowski TJ, Pollen AA, Sandoval-Espinosa C, et al. Transformation of the radial glia scaffold demarcates two stages of human cerebral cortex development. Neuron. 2016;**91**:1219-1227

[47] Taniguchi-Ikeda M, Koyanagi-Aoi M, Maruyama T, et al. Restoration of the defect in radial glial fiber migration and cortical plate organization in a brain organoid model of Fukuyama muscular dystrophy. 2021;**24**:103140

[48] Qian X, Su Y, Adam CD, et al. Sliced human cortical organoids for modeling distinct cortical layer formation. Cell Stem Cell. 2020;**26**:766-781.e9

[49] Long KR, Newland B, Florio M, et al. Extracellular matrix components HAPLN1, Lumican, and collagen I cause hyaluronic acid-dependent folding of the developing human neocortex. Neuron. 2018;**99**:702-719.e6

[50] Garcez PP, Loiola EC, Madeiro da Costa R, et al. Zika virus impairs

growth in human neurospheres and brain organoids. Science. *1979*;**2016**(352):816-818

[51] Camp JG, Badsha F, Florio M, et al. Human cerebral organoids recapitulate gene expression programs of fetal neocortex development. Proceedings of the National Academy of Sciences of the United States of America. 2015;**112**:15672-15677

[52] Pavlinek A, Adhya D, Tsompanidis A, et al. Using organoids to model sex differences in the human brain. Biological Psychiatry Global Open Science. 2024;**4**:100343

[53] Hanzlik E, Gigante J. Microcephaly. Children (Basel). 2017;**4**:47

[54] Javed AO, Li Y, Muffat J, et al. Microcephaly modeling of kinetochore mutation reveals a brain-specific phenotype. Cell Reports. 2018;**25**:368-382

[55] Yoon K-J, Song G, Qian X, et al. Zika-virus-encoded NS2A disrupts mammalian cortical neurogenesis by degrading adherens junction proteins. Cell Stem Cell. 2017;**21**:349-358

[56] Smirnova L, Hartung T. The promise and potential of brain organoids. Advanced Healthcare Materials. 2024;**13**:1-11

[57] Dixon TA, Muotri AR. Advancing preclinical models of psychiatric disorders with human brain organoid cultures. Molecular Psychiatry. 2023;**28**:83-95

[58] Schafer ST, Paquola ACM, Stern S, et al. Pathological priming causes developmental gene network heterochronicity in autistic subject-derived neurons. Nature Neuroscience. 2019;**22**:243-255

[59] Lu X, Yang J, Xiang Y. Modeling human neurodevelopmental diseases with brain organoids. Cell Regeneration. 2022;**11**:1

[60] Colantuoni C, Jeon O-H, Hyder K, et al. Gene expression profiling in postmortem Rett syndrome brain: Differential gene expression and patient classification. Neurobiology of Disease. 2001;**8**:847-865

[61] Chen RZ, Akbarian S, Tudor M, et al. Deficiency of methyl-CpG binding protein-2 in CNS neurons results in a Rett-like phenotype in mice. Nature Genetics. 2001;**27**:327-331

[62] Haase FD, Coorey B, Riley L, et al. Pre-clinical investigation of Rett syndrome using human stem cell-based disease models. Frontiers in Neuroscience. 2021;**15**:698812

[63] Han D, Xue X, Yan Y, et al. Highlight article: Dysfunctional Cav1.2 channel in Timothy syndrome, from cell to bedside. Experimental Biology and Medicine. 2019;**244**:960

[64] Xu R, Brawner AT, Li S, et al. OLIG2 drives abnormal neurodevelopmental phenotypes in human iPSC-based organoid and chimeric mouse models of down syndrome. Cell Stem Cell. 2019;**24**:908-926

[65] Romero-Morales AI, Robertson GL, Rastogi A, et al. Human iPSC-derived cerebral organoids model features of Leigh syndrome and reveal abnormal corticogenesis. Development. 2022;**149**(20):dev199914

[66] Wray S. Seminars in cell and developmental biology modelling neurodegenerative disease using brain organoids. Seminars in Cell & Developmental Biology. 2021;**111**:60-66

[67] Babu HW, Kumar SM, Kaur H, et al. Midbrain organoids for Parkinson's disease (PD)-A powerful tool to understand the disease pathogenesis. Life Sciences. 2024;**345**:122610

[68] Raja WK, Mungenast AE, Lin Y-T, et al. Self-organizing 3D human neural tissue derived from induced pluripotent stem cells recapitulate Alzheimer's disease phenotypes. PLoS One. 2016;**11**:e0161969

[69] Paşca SP, Portmann T, Voineagu I, et al. Using iPSC-derived neurons to uncover cellular phenotypes associated with Timothy syndrome. Nature Medicine. 2011;**17**:1657-1662

[70] Hartung T, Morales Pantoja IE, Smirnova L. Brain organoids and organoid intelligence from ethical, legal, and social points of view. Frontiers in Artificial Intelligence. 2024;**6**:1307613

[71] Sun XY, Ju XC, Li Y, et al. Generation of vascularized brain organoids to study neurovascular interactions. 2022;**11**:e76707

[72] Maheshwari S, Akram H, Bulstrode H, et al. Dopaminergic cell replacement for Parkinson's disease: Addressing the intracranial delivery hurdle. Journal of Parkinson's Disease. 2024;**14**:415-435

[73] Tabar V, Sarva H, Lozano AM, et al. Phase I trial of hES cell-derived dopaminergic neurons for Parkinson's disease. Nature. *2025*;**2025**(11):1-6

[74] Pereira A, Diwakar J, Masserdotti G, et al. Direct neuronal reprogramming of mouse astrocytes is associated with multiscale epigenome remodeling and requires Yy1. Nature Neuroscience. 2024;**27**:1260-1273

[75] Dennison R, Usuga E, Chen H, et al. Direct cell reprogramming and phenotypic conversion: An analysis of experimental attempts to transform astrocytes into neurons in adult animals. Cells. 2023;**12**:618

[76] Yuan M, Tang Y, Huang T, et al. In situ direct reprogramming of astrocytes to neurons via polypyrimidine tract-binding protein 1 knockdown in a mouse model of ischemic stroke. Neural Regeneration Research. 2024;**19**:2240-2248

[77] Lee CT, Bendriem RM, Wu WW, et al. 3D brain organoids derived from pluripotent stem cells: Promising experimental models for brain development and neurodegenerative disorders. Journal of Biomedical Science. 2017;**24**:1-12

[78] Andrews MG, Kriegstein AR. Challenges of organoid research. Annual Review of Neuroscience. 2022;**45**:23-39

[79] Kim SH, Chang MY. Application of human brain organoids—Opportunities and challenges in modeling human brain development and neurodevelopmental diseases. International Journal of Molecular Sciences. 2023;**24**:12528

[80] Kataoka M, Lee TL, Sawai T. Human brain organoid research and applications: Where and how to meet legal challenges? Journal of Bioethical Inquiry. 2024;**21**:603-610

[81] Nature Reviews Bioengineering (Editorial). Ethics need to keep up with human brain organoid research. Nature Reviews Bioengineering. 2024;**2**:711

[82] Jang H, Kim SH, Koh Y, et al. Engineering brain organoids: Toward mature neural circuitry with an intact Cytoarchitecture. International Journal of Stem Cells. 2022;**15**:41-59

[83] Xu Z, Li E, Guo Z, et al. Design and construction of a multi-organ

microfluidic chip mimicking the in vivo microenvironment of lung cancer metastasis. ACS Applied Materials & Interfaces. 2016;**8**:25840-25847

[84] Koyanagi M, Ogido R, Moriya A, et al. Development of a 3-dimensional organotypic model with characteristics of peripheral sensory nerves. Cell Reports Methods. 2024;**4**:100835

[85] Kim J, Imaizumi K, Jurjuț O, et al. Human assembloid model of the ascending neural sensory pathway. Nature. 2025;**642**:143-153

[86] Zheng T, Wu L, Sun S, et al. Co-culture of Schwann cells and endothelial cells for synergistically regulating dorsal root ganglion behavior on chitosan-based anisotropic topology for peripheral nerve regeneration. Burns & Trauma. 2022;**10**:tkac030

[87] Pereira JD, DuBreuil DM, Devlin AC, et al. Human sensorimotor organoids derived from healthy and amyotrophic lateral sclerosis stem cells form neuromuscular junctions. Nature Communications. 2021;**12**:1-17

[88] Bendriem RM, Singh S, Aleem AA, et al. Tight junction protein occludin regulates progenitor self-renewal and survival in developing cortex. Elife. 2019;**8**:e49376

[89] Wang P, Mokhtari R, Pedrosa E, et al. CRISPR/Cas9-mediated heterozygous knockout of the autism gene CHD8 and characterization of its transcriptional networks in cerebral organoids derived from iPS cells. Molecular Autism. 2017;**8**:1-17

[90] Smirnova L, Caffo BS, Gracias DH, et al. Organoid intelligence (OI): The new frontier in biocomputing and intelligence-in-a-dish. Frontiers in Science. 2023;**1**:1017235

[91] Kagan BJ, Kitchen AC, Tran NT, et al. In vitro neurons learn and exhibit sentience when embodied in a simulated game-world. Neuron. 2022;**110**:3952-3969.e8

[92] Lewis J, Holm S. Regulating organoid and organoid-related activities: An analysis of the regulatory gaps and areas of over-regulation. HYBRIDA. 2022;**75**

[93] Hyun I, Scharf-Deering JC, Lunshof JE. Ethical issues related to brain organoid research. Brain Research. 2020;**1732**:146653

[94] Lavazza A, Massimini M. Cerebral organoids: Ethical issues and consciousness assessment. Journal of Medical Ethics. 2018;**44**:606-610

[95] Hermerén G. Ethical considerations in chimera research. Development. 2015;**142**:3-5

[96] Kreitmair K. Consciousness and the ethics of human brain organoid research. Cambridge Quarterly of Healthcare Ethics. 2023;**32**:518-528

[97] Jeziorski J, Brandt R, Evans JH, et al. Brain organoids, consciousness, ethics and moral status. Seminars in Cell & Developmental Biology. 2023;**144**:97-102

[98] 3. Clinical Translation of Stem Cell-based Interventions—International Society for Stem Cell Research. Available from: https://www.isscr.org/guidelines/blog-post-title-one-ed2td-6fcdk-5zr5l [Accessed: 6 June 2025]

Chapter 4

Molecular Analysis of Chinese FOXG1-Related Encephalopathy

Guanting Lu, Gang Mai and Qiongling Peng

Abstract

FOXG1-related encephalopathy, also referred to as FOXG1-related disease or FOXG1 syndrome, impacts the majority of developmental elements and results in brain abnormalities and microcephaly. This syndrome was categorized as a congenital variant of Rett syndrome. The primary cause of this disorder was thought to be the aberrant expression or function of the *FOXG1* gene, which was resulted from intragenic mutations, microduplications or microdeletions. As of right now, most FOXG1-related encephalopathies have been found in North America and Europe, with very few instances documented in China. Till now, only 17 Chinese cases were reported. Some clinical features could be seen in almost all cases, including delayed language development, seizures, feeding difficulties, and corpus callosum hypoplasia, as well as underdevelopment of the temporal and frontal lobes. Four patients (23.53%) exhibited copy number variations (CNVs) affecting *FOXG1* (1 microduplication and 3 microdeletions), while 13 patients (76.47%) had single-nucleotide mutations of the *FOXG1* gene. CNVs in several brain-active regulatory elements located in the intergenic region between *FOXG1* and *PRKD1* (FOXG1-PRKD1) may possibly potentially disrupt FOXG1 expression. Subsequent research suggested that *PRKD1* could work in concert to modulate the relationships of *CDKL5*, *MECP2*, and *FOXG1*, which could lead to the development of RTT/RTT-like disorders. The molecular etiology of FOXG1-related illnesses would be better understood thanks to this reanalysis, which would also aid with future gene therapy, diagnostics, and treatment. This re-analysis would expand the current understanding of molecular etiology and contribute to the future diagnosis, treatment, as well as gene therapy of FOXG1-related disorders.

Keywords: Rett syndrome, FOXG1-related encephalopathy, copy number variation, intergenic, PRKD1, regulatory elements

1. Introduction

Rett syndrome (RTT; OMIM#312750) is a severe neurodevelopmental syndrome affecting ~1/10,000 females. It is primarily caused by *MECP2* (OMIM#300005) mutations, accounting for about 90% of cases, and follows an XLD inheritance pattern [1, 2]. Early growth arrest (often 6–18 months postpartum), hand stereotypies, delayed acquisition of skills, loss of language, microcephaly, varying intellectual impairment (ID), and seizures are among the clinical phenotypes that have been described [3]. According to reports, around 90% of RTT cases result from mutations in the MECP2 gene. In addition to *MECP2*, the gene *FOXG1* [4] has also been linked to RTT or RTT-like diseases as genetic factors.

Patients carrying pathogenic *FOXG1* mutations were characterized by congenital microcephaly, corpus callosum hypoplasia, and severe intellectual disability, emerging as a distinct entity from classical RTT due to three key differences. (1) earlier onset: Symptoms arise prenatally or within the first 6 months of life, contrasting with RTT's postnatal regression (~6–18 months) [5]; (2) unique phenotypes: Patients exhibit profound hypotonia, lack of purposeful hand movements, and minimal language acquisition, without the characteristic RTT hand stereotypies [5, 6]; (3) molecular divergence: It could be caused by multiple types of mutations, for instance, single-nucleotide variants, microdeletions, and even microduplication leading to increasing expression of FOXG1. Therefore, the disorder associated with FOXG1 mutations was termed as "FOXG1-related encephalopathy" [7], "FOXG1-related disorder" [8], or "FOXG1-related syndrome" [9].

FOXG1, as fork-head transcription repressor, has strong expression in neural systems, including the olfactory placodes, nasal retina, otic vesicles, and telencephalon. In vertebrates, it is a characteristic of the telencephalon [10]. It is crucial for the growth of the corpus callosum, cerebral cortex, and telencephalon [11]. The formation of the neuronal GABAergic inhibitory circuit depends critically on the *FOXG1* expression level at a particular developmental stage. In mouse models, its aberrant expression led to ASD-like social deficits and was harmful to the development of the inhibitory circuit [12]. Additionally, it is crucial for the pacing of telencephalic neurogenesis and the patterning of the early rostral brain, particularly for promoting dendritic elongation [13]. Despite modulating the neurological development of telencephalon during embryogenesis, FOXG1 expression persists postnatally and throughout adulthood for preventing apoptosis and enhancing postmitotic neuronal survival [14], maintaining neuroplasticity [15], and encouraging the development of the hippocampus dentate gyrus, particularly in the early postnatal stage [16], all of which are essential for high-grade function.

Currently, about 259 patients have been identified as carriers of 161 specific pathogenic mutations within the coding sequence (CDS) of the FOXG1 [5, 6, 17–19], including 61 (37.89, 61/161) frameshifts, 34 (21.12%, 34/161) nonsenses, 4 (2.48%) in-frame deletions, and 67 (41.64%, 67/161) missenses. Among these mutations, the first two kinds were distributed along the CDS, the missense mutations were almost located within the DNA-binding forkhead domain (FHD, 181–269), with one additional mutation (p.Ser393Trp) occurring in the JARID1B-binding domain (JBD, 383–406). Since FOXG1 is a single exon gene, transcripts with truncating variants (frameshifts and nonsenses) may evade nonsense-mediated decay (NMD), thereby encoding truncated proteins that could affect the severity of clinical phenotypes. Patients harboring truncating mutations but retaining the DNA-binding FHD domain (aa 181–269) were contrasted with those with N-terminal truncating variants (aa 1–275). Those with C-terminal truncating mutations were more likely to have some specific gross or fine motor abilities, and autism spectrum disorders (ASDs). This displayed that retaining the DNA-binding FHD domain might be important for the variable severity of phenotypes.

Despite progresses in elucidating *FOXG1*'s role in neuronal development [7], the molecular mechanisms underlying its pathogenesis remain poorly understood, especially for non-European populations. Only 17 cases of FOXG1-related disorders have been identified in Chinese patients since the first reported case of FOXG1 gene mutation in China in 2017.

2. Comprehensive analysis of 17 cases of FOXG1 gene mutation in Chinese patients

Up to now, only 17 cases have been documented in China, all carrying 17 *de novo* FOXG1 gene mutations [2, 20]. The clinical characteristics and medical records of all patients were meticulously gathered and analyzed in order to obtain a thorough analysis for these mutations (**Table 1**). The patients were ranked based on the site of mutation on the FOXG1 protein. When the clinical characteristics of 17 patients were compiled, 11 of them (64.71%) were female and just 6 (35.29%) were male. Fourteen patients (82.35%, 14/17) had the phenotype of microcephaly. Three patients (17.65%, 3/17) had regression, which is the gradual loss of motor skills or acquired language. Four patients were also found to have bruxism. Regarding musculoskeletal system, nearly all patients had stereotypic and hypotonia motions with the limited functional hand usage. No patient was able to walk or sit normally at early stages, but as they grew older, six of them were able to sit without assistance after 10 months. As for the eyes, almost all of the patients suffered from difficulties in maintaining eye contact and were unable to track moving objects.

Regarding central nervous system (CNS) phenotypes, the majority of individuals had feeding difficulties, delayed speech, abnormal EEG, and seizures. The first-recorded onset period for seizures was 4 months or later. There have been reports of both partial and generalized tonic-clonic seizures. The majority of the patients had underdeveloped temporal and frontal lobes and hypoplasia of the corpus callosum, according to MRI. Four cases of hypomyelination or delayed myelination were reported.

3. Single-nucleotide mutations identified in Chinese patients

The mapping of *FOXG1* gene to human genome reference was performed using UCSC genome browser. The gene was located within an evolutionarily conserved region (**Figure 1A**) and comprised a single exon (**Figure 1B**). So far, 13 heterozygous mutations were detected in Chinese patients to impair the protein coding-sequence. Among these *de novo* mutations, there were two missenses, four nonsenses, and seven frameshift mutations.

As for these mutations, c.460dup (p.Glu154GlyfsTer301, rs398124204, patient 3) has been reported over 10 times in European patients [6, 29–37], but only once in Chinese patients [21]. Two patients with Rett syndrome in China were identified as carriers of the c.506dup mutation (rs1450095073, Patient 3), while the other two patients carried frameshift mutations (patient 6: c.974dup; patient 5: c.858dup) [21, 22]. The open-reading frames with these four frameshifting mutations all terminate at the same termination codon, causing the production of a truncated protein containing 455 amino acids, despite their differing replication sites (**Figure 1F**). The functions of enlarged region were unknown.

Additionally, two missense mutations were found in the DNA-binding FHD (c.590G > T, p.Ser197Ile in patient 6 and c.694A > T, p.Asn232Tyr in case 8). Asn232 and Ser197 were both highly evolutionarily conserved amino acids (**Figure 1-D**). They were rated as "likely pathogenic" in accordance with the ACMG criterion categories (**Table 1**). Additionally, this mutation causes the exposed Ile (26.6%) to replace the buried Ser (RSA 2.3%) (**Figure 1G-H**). The local structure of the PHD domain may be disturbed by the buried/exposed switch and the buried H-bond breakdown. The side

General information	**Lu et al. [2]**	**Zhang et al. [21]**	**Niu et al. [22]**	**Bai et al. [23]**	**Zhang et al. [21]**	**Zhang et al. [21]**	**Bai et al. [23]**	**Zhang et al. [21]**	**Bai et al. [23]**
Patient No.	Patient 1	Patient 2	Patient 3	Patient 4	Patient 5	Patient 6	Patient 7	Patient 8	Patient 9
Sex	Female	Female	Female	Female	Female	Female	Female	Female	Female
Age	23 m	12 m	2 y 5 m	18 m	4.5 y	20 m	2 m	2 y	30 m
Molecular characterization									
Locations (hg19)	14:29236870	14:29236945	14:29236986	14:29237075	14:29237179	14:29237343	14:29237408	14:29237457	14:29128665–30,217,058
Genetic mutations	c.385G > T (p.Glu129Ter)	c.460dup (p. Glu154GlyfsTer301)	c.506dup (p. Lys170GlnfsTer285)	c.590G > T (p.Ser197Ile)	c.694A > T (p. Asn232Tyr)	c.858dup (p. Lys287GlnfsTer168)	c.923G > A (p. Trp308Ter)	c.974dup (p. Leu325PhefsTer130)	/
CMAs	/	/	/	/	/	/	/	/	arr[hg19]14q12 (29128665–30,217,058)x1
Consequence	Stopgain	Frameshift	Frameshift	Missense	Missense	Frameshift	Stopgain	Frameshift	Microdeletion
Karyotypes	46, XX	46, XX	46, XX	46, XX	46, XX	46, XX	46, XX	46, XX	46, XX, del(14)(q12)
ACMG classification	Pathogenic PVS1 + PS2 + PM2	Pathogenic PVS1 + PS2 + PM2	Pathogenic PVS1 + PS2 + PM2	Likely Pathogenic PM1 + PM2 + PP2 + PP3 + PP5	Likely Pathogenic PS2 + PM2 + PP3	Pathogenic PVS1 + PS2 + PM2	Pathogenic PVS1 + PM2 + PP5	Pathogenic PVS1 + PS2 + PM2	/
dbSNP ID	rs1555321264	rs398124204	rs1452295073	rs1881802605	rs786205486	/	/	/	/
Inheritance	*de novo*	*de novo*	*de novo*	*de novo*	*de novo*	*de novo*	*de novo*	*de novo*	*de novo*
Head OFC (cm)	42	43	40.5	39	49	42	38.5	45.5	/
Microcephaly	Y	Y	Y	Y	N	Y	Y	Y	/
Regression	N	N	Y	N	N	Y	N	N	Y
Bruxism	Y	Y, 12 m	/	/	Y, 12 m	Y, 19 m	/	N	/
Motor development									
Stereotypic movements	Y	Y, 3 m	Y	Y	Y, 10 m	Y, 12 m	Y	Y, 8 m	Y
Limited hand use	Y	Y	/	Y	Y	Y	Y	Y	Y
Rising head (Age)	Y,10 m	Y, 8 m	Y, 11 m	Y	Y, 5 m	Y, 7 m	Y	Y, 2 m	Y,9 m
Sitting	N	N	N	Y	Y, 12 m	N	Y	Y, 10 m	Y,11 m

General information	Lu et al. [2]	Zhang et al. [21]	Niu et al. [22]	Bai et al. [23]	Zhang et al. [21]	Zhang et al. [21]	Bai et al. [23]	Zhang et al. [21]	Bai et al. [23]
Walking	N	N	N	N	N, standing with aid at 24 m	N	N	N	N
Poor eye contact	Y	Y	Y	Y	Y	/	Y	Y	Y
Central nervous system									
Hypotonia	Y	Y	Y	Y	Y	Y	Y	Y	Y
Delayed speech	Y	Y	Y	Y	Y	Y	Y	Y	Y
Feeding difficulties	Y	Y	Y	/	Y	/	/	Y	/
EEG abnormalities	Y	Y	Y	N	Y	Y	N	Y	N
Seizure onset time (Age)	Y, 18 m	Y, 10 m	Y, 16 m	N	Y, 6 m	Y, 10.5 m	N	Y, 10.5 m	Y, 13-15 m
Seizure types	Generalized tonic-clonic	Partial	Generalized tonic-clonic	N	Partial	Partial	N	Partial	/
Seizure with cyanosis	N	Y	/	N	Y	Y	N	Y	Y
Sleep disturbances	Y	Y	Y	/	Y	N	/	Y	/
Corpus callosum hypoplasia	Y	Y	Y	N	Y	Y	N	Y	N
Delayed myelination or hypomyelination	Y	N	N	N	N	Y	N	N	N
Underdevelopment of frontal and temporal lobes	Y	Y	Y	Y	Y	Y	Y	Y, mild	Y

General information	Li et al. [24]	Tang et al. [25]	Wang et al. [26]	Hu et al. [20]	Cui et al. [27]	Sun et al. [28]	Sun et al. [28]	Sun et al. [28]
Patient No.	Patient 10	Patient 11	Patient 12	Patient 13	Patient 14	Patient 15	Patient 16	Patient 17
Sex	Male	Female	Female	Male	Male	Male	Male	Male
Age	8 d	3 y	9y	3 m	5 m	16 m	5y	3y6m
Molecular characterization								
Locations (hg19)	14:25084632–34,690,056	14:26622393–31,444,468	14:28904992–30,805,462	14:29237003	14:29237640	14:29236741	14:29237080	14:29237663
Genetic mutations	/	/	/	c.518delA (p. Glu173GlyfsTer19)	c.1155insT (p. Ala386CysfsTer35)	c.256dup (p. Gln86ProfsTer35)	c.595G > T (p. Glu199Ter)	c.1178C > A (p. Ser393Ter)

General information	Li et al. [24]	Tang et al. [25]	Wang et al. [26]	Hu et al. [20]	Cui et al. [27]	Sun et al. [28]	Sun et al. [28]	Sun et al. [28]
CMAs	arr[hg19]14q12q13.1 (25084632–4,690,056)x1	arr[hg19]14q12 (26622393–31,444,468)x1	arr[hg19]14q12 (28904992–30,805,462)x3	/	/	/	/	/
Consequence	Microdeletion	Microdeletion	Microduplication	/	/	/	/	/
Karyotypes	46, XY, del(14)(q12q13.1)	46, XX, del(14)(q12)	46, XX, dup(14)(q12)	46, XX,	46, XX,	46, XX,	46, XX,	46, XX,
ACMG classification	/	/	/	PVS1 + PM2 + PS2	PVS1 + PS2 + PM2	PVS1 + PS2 + PM2	PVS1 + PS2 + PM2	PVS1 + PS2 + PM2
dbSNP ID	/	/	/	/	/	rs786205001	/	rs1085307753
Inheritance	*de novo*	*de novo*	*de novo*	*de novo*	*de novo*	*de novo*	*de novo*	*de novo*
Head OFC (cm)	/	/	46	/	/	/	/	/
Microcephaly	/	/	Y	/	/	Y	Y	Y
Regression	/	/	/	/	/	N	N	N
Bruxism	/	/	/	/	/	/	/	/
Motor development								
Stereotypic movements	/	/	Y	/	Y	Y	Y	N
Limited hand use	/	/	Y	Y	Y	Y	Y	Y
Rising head (Age)	/	/	Y, 36 m	N	N	Y, 6 m		Y
Sitting	/	/	Y, 48 m	N	N	N	Y	Y
Walking	/	/	Y,72 m	N	N	NA	N	N
Poor eye contact	/	Y	Y	Y	Y	Y	Y	Y
Central nervous system								
Hypotonia	Y, 8 d	/	Y	Y	Y	Y	Y	Y
Delayed speech	/	Y	Y	Y	Y	Y	Y	Y
Feeding difficulties	Y, 8 d	/	Y	/	/	/	Y	/
EEG abnormalities	/	Y	Y	/	/	N	/	/
Seizure onset time (Age)	/	Y,?	Y, 4 m	/	/	Y,16 m	N	/
Seizure types	/	?	?	/	/	/	N	/

General information	Li et al. [24]	Tang et al. [25]	Wang et al. [26]	Hu et al. [20]	Cui et al. [27]	Sun et al. [28]	Sun et al. [28]	Sun et al. [28]
Seizure with cyanosis	/	/	/	/	/	/	N	/
Sleep disturbances	/	/	/	/	/	Y	Y	/
Corpus callosum hypoplasia	Y	/	Y	Y	Y	Y	Y	Y
Delayed myelination or hypomyelination	/	/	/	/	Y	Y	/	Y
Underdevelopment of frontal and temporal lobes	/	/	Y	Y	/	Y	Y	/

Table 1.
Clinical information of the 17 FOXG1-related disorders.

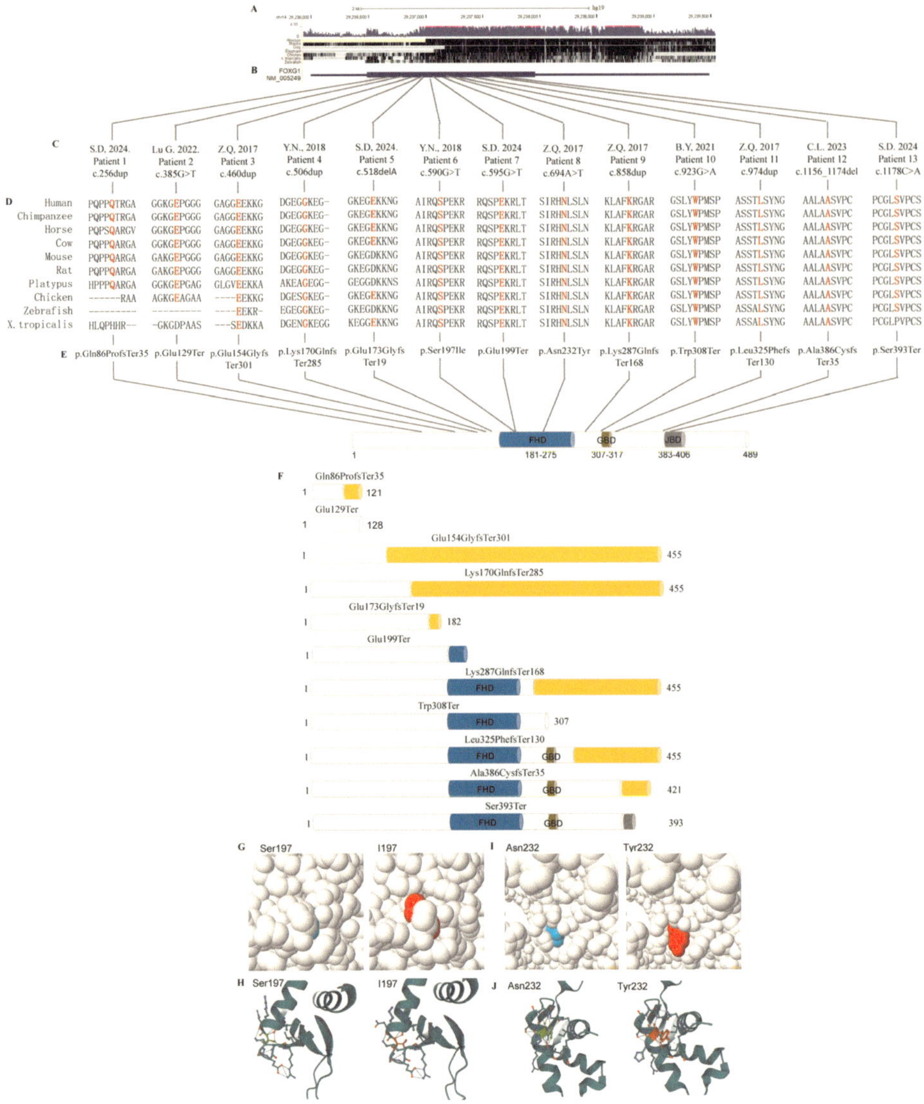

Figure 1.
FOXG1 gene single-nucleotide mutations detected in Chinese patients. (A) Conservation of the genomic region; (B) FOXG1 gene structure; (C) nucleotide variations in mutations; (D) conservation analysis of the mutations; (E) amino acid variations in mutations; (F) proteins with truncating mutations. (G) FHD domain structure with Ser197; (H) FHD domain structure with Ile197; (I) FHD domain structure with N232; (J) FHD domain structure with Y232. The yellow cylinder indicates abnormal amino acids resulting from frameshifting mutations (Adopted from Lu et al. [2]).

chain of Tyr (Y) is a bulky p-hydroxyphenyl, whereas that of Asn (N) is a small-sized aminocarbonyl for c.694A > T (p.Asn232Tyr). According to Missense3D analysis, this mutation caused all side-chain/side-chain H-bonds to be broken by changing from a buried Asn (RSA 7.0%) to an exposed Tyr (63.4%). Tyr232 creates only one side-chain/main-chain hydrogen bond with Asn236 (AO236-Asn ND2/AO232-Tyr O) (**Figure 1I-J**). These molecular changing might affect the DNA-binding ability of the FHD domain.

Variants designated as "Likely Pathogenic" and "Pathogenic" from DECIPTHER and NCBI ClinVar were compared to the CDS of *FOXG1* for thoroughly investigating the mutation patterns of *FOXG1*. In both databases, a total of 171 mutations in the *FOXG1* CDS were found. The mutation may be categorized as initiator loss, frameshift, missense, stop-gain (or nonsense), or terminator loss. These mutations were found in various *FOXG1* functional domains [7]. Missense (38.60%, 66/171) and frameshift (37.43%, 64/171) were accounted for most of the mutation types. Nonsense mutations were the third most common types (23.98%, 41/171). About 93.94% (62/66) of the missense mutations were found in the DNA-binding FHD domain, and 4.55% (3/66) were found in the JBD, which is in charge of the interaction between JARID1B (also known as KDM5B) and FOXG1. The C-terminal disordered region contains a single missense (c.1439A > G, p.Gln480Arg) with an uncertain function. The pathogenic duplications and deletions (dup/del) were found over the entire FOXG1 reading-frame. Since the *FOXG1* gene only has one exon, transcripts with frameshift or nonsense mutations may translate into abnormal proteins rather than being degraded by NMD [38]. The diversity of mutation types and sites may influence the expression levels of functionally normal FOXG1, potentially representing the potential molecular mechanism for the diversity of clinical manifestations in encephalopathies linked to FOXG1.

4. CNVs containing *FOXG1* gene

Among Chinese patients, four distinct CNVs were identified, comprising one microduplication and three microdeletions (**Table 1**). Regarding the three microdeletions (Li.S_2021, Tang.Z_2021, and Bai.Y_2021), the shortest one (Bai.Y_2021, 14:29128665-30,217,058, 1.09 Mb) covered only two genes, *FOXG1* and *PRKD1* (**Figure 2A-B**) [23]. The microduplication identified at 14q12 (14:27974743-29,875,213, 1.90 Mb) contained only the *FOXG1* gene [26].

Approximately 76 independent deletion fragments covering the Li.S_2021 genomic region (chromosome 14: 25,084,632–34,690,056) were collected from multiple public databases, encompassing 21 in ClinVar, 10 in ClinGen (Clinical Genome Resource), 29 in the Copy Number Variation Morbidity Map of Developmental Delay and Intellectual Disability (DD/ID), and 16 in DECIPHER [39, 40] databases (**Figure 2C-F**). Out of these microdeletions, 31 (40.79%) covered the whole region of FOXG1 gene. Six short deletions only contained the *FOXG1* gene, where three shortest deletions, 290,100 (chr14: 29,236,278-29,237,804, 1.52Kb, DECIPHER), 820,618 (chr14: 29,236,466-29,237,975, 1.51Kb, ClinVar), as well as 1,057,648 (chr14: 29,236,486-29,237,955, 1.47Kb, ClinVar) only covered the protein-coding sequence of *FOXG1. FOXG1* should be the key molecular factor for neurodevelopmental diseases with 14q12 anomalies since it has been shown to be necessary for the development of the telencephalon, synaptic plasticity, postmitotic neuron survival, as well as the establishment of the hippocampal dentate gyrus.

5. PRKD1 related to neurodevelopmental disorders

The *PRKD1* gene was identified as the molecular etiology of CHDED since it is the downstream gene next to FOXG1 (OMIM#617364) [41]. Information on pathogenic mutations in the CDS of *PRKD1* was integrated from DECIPHER and ClinVar

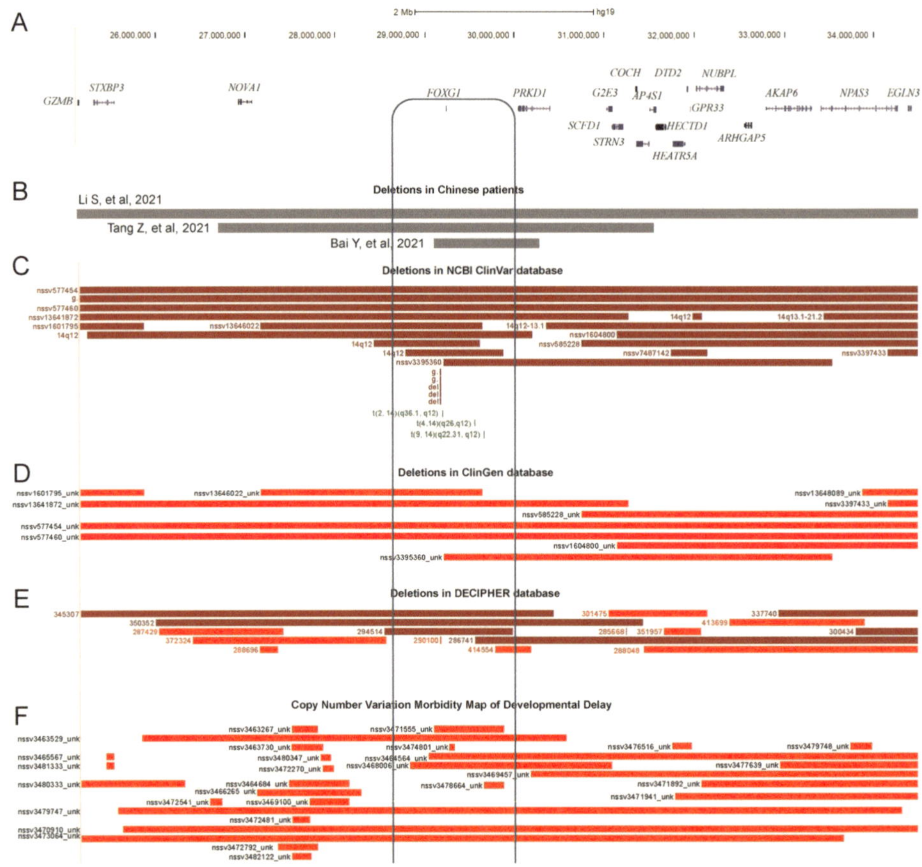

Figure 2.

Characteristic analysis of FOXG1 gene microdeletions. (A) Protein coding genes and genomic regions of microdeletion in patients 9, 10, and 11; (B) microdeletion-covered regions in two Chinese patients; (C) microdeletions in ClinGen database, (D) NCBI's ClinVar database, (E) DECIPHER database (F) developmental delay, and (G) database of genomic variants (DGVs) (adopted from Lu et al. [2]).

databases, along with the published articles. Single-nucleotide variants identified as pathogenic or likely pathogenic were determined in 20 cases (**Figure 3A** and **Table 2**). Ten were homozygous (from four distinct consanguineous families) and 10 were heterozygous (1 unknown and 9 *de novo*). It is important to note after gathering the clinical characteristics of these individuals that all of the patients with homozygous mutations had congenital heart disorders (CHDs) and no other systemic abnormalities [42–44]. This was in line with the phenotypes in mice with homozygous *Prkd1* deletion. The mice exhibited complicated forms of CHD, including bicuspid aortic and pulmonary valves and atrioventricular septal abnormalities [45]. It is surprising that heterozygous mutations may cause CHDs as well as abnormalities in the CNS, including hearing impairment, delayed language development, global developmental delay, intellectual disability, and microcephaly [41, 46].

Additionally, the DECIPHER and ClinVar databases have documented some CNVs that partially or fully cover the PRKD1 gene (9 microdeletions and 5 microduplications) (**Figure 3B**). The remaining 10 CNVs—1 microduplication and 9 microdeletions—were submitted to further study, with the exception of 4 microduplications that lacked the clinical characteristics. In addition to cardiovascular

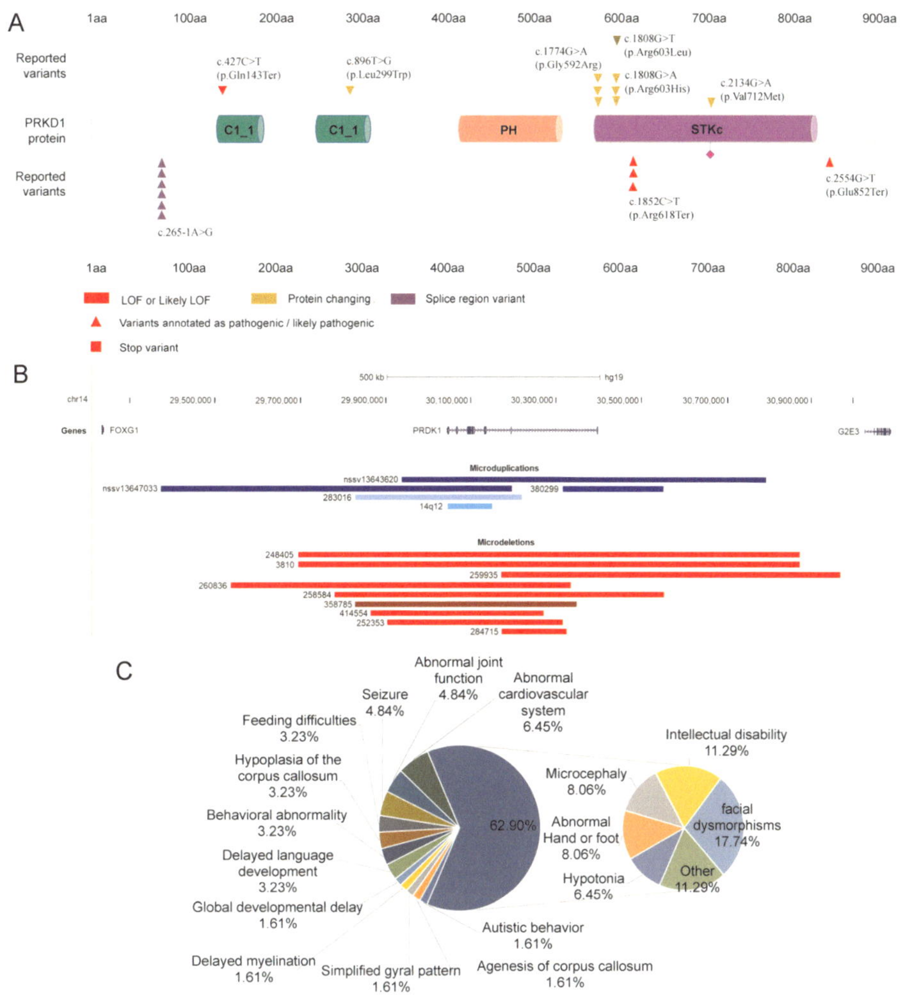

Figure 3.
Distribution of PRKD1 gene mutations. (A) Distribution of SNMs in PRKD1; (B) CNVs of PRKD1; (C) proportion of clinical phenotypes among individuals with CNVs containing PRKD1 (Adopted from Lu et al. [2]).

abnormalities (hypertension, ventricular septal defect, Tetralogy of Fallot) present in 6.45% (4/62) of the 62 reported clinical phenotypes, there were also RTT-like phenotypes, for instance, agenesis of corpus callosum (1.61%, 1/62), global developmental delay (1.61%, 1/62), simplified gyral pattern (1.61%, 1/62), delayed myelination (1.61%, 1/62), delayed language development (3.23%, 2/62), hypoplasia of the corpus callosum (3.23%, 2/62), feeding difficulties (3.23%, 2/62), behavioral abnormality (3.23%, 2/62), seizures (4.84%, 3/62), hypotonia (6.45%, 4/62), microcephaly (8.06%, 5/62), intellectual disability (11.29%, 7/62), facial dysmorphisms (17.74%, 11/62), as well as others (11.29%, 7/62) (**Figure 3C**). Other symptoms included intra-uterine growth restriction, hypothyroidism, bruxism, obesity, nystagmus, microdontia, and short stature.

The *PRKD1* gene was covered in two microdeletions identified in two Chinese patients. Patients that had heterozygous mutations or CNVs affecting the *PRKD1* gene had global developmental delay, intellectual disability, delayed language development,

No.	Patient	Sex	Gene	Location (GRCh37)	Reference	Nucleotide	Amino acid	SNP ID	Consequence	Pathogenicity/ contribution	Zygosity	CHD classification	Phenotypes	PMID
1	261,674 (Patient 1)	46XY	PRKD1	14:30107911	NM_002742	c.896 T > G	p. Leu299Trp	rs1057519636	Missense	Likely pathogenic PM2 + PP3 + PS2 + PP4	*De novo* heterozygous	Syndromic	Arnold-Chiari type I malformation; atrioventricular canal defect; attention deficit hyperactivity disorder; microcephaly; nystagmus; specific learning disability	27,479,907
2	263,568 (Patient 3)	46XY	PRKD1	14:30095714	NM_002742	c.1774G > A	p. Gly592Arg	rs1057519635	Missense	Likely pathogenic	*De novo* heterozygous	Syndromic	2–3 toe syndactyly; abnormal cardiac septum morphology; Abnormality of prenatal development or birth; brachycephaly; Deep plantar creases; depressed nasal bridge; finger syndactyly; fragile nails; frontal bossing; generalized hypotonia; high anterior hairline; hypoplasia of teeth; melanocytic nevus; scoliosis; sparse scalp hair; stridor; thin skin	27,479,907
3	268,276 (Patient 2)	46XY	PRKD1	14:30095714	NM_002742	c.1774G > A	p. Gly592Arg	rs1057519635	Missense	Pathogenic	*De novo* heterozygous	Syndromic	bilateral conductive hearing impairment; broad thumb; delayed speech and language	27,479,907

No.	Patient	Sex	Gene	Location (GRCh37)	Reference	Nucleotide	Amino acid	SNP ID	Consequence	Pathogenicity/ contribution	Zygosity	CHD classification	Phenotypes	PMID
													development; dry skin; premature loss of primary teeth; pulmonic stenosis; short digit; sparse scalp hair	
4	272,461	46XY	PRKD1	14:30135391	NM_002742	c.427C > T	p. Gln143Ter	/	Stop gain	Pathogenic	Unknown heterozygous	Syndromic	depressed nasal bridge; hypotonia; moderate global developmental delay; protruding tongue; synophrys	/
5	413,370	46XX	PRKD1	14:30093455	NM_002742	c.1808G > A	p. Arg603His	rs776034417	Missense	Likely pathogenic PM2 + PP3 + PS2	*De novo* heterozygous	Syndromic	Atrioventricular canal defect; cleft palate; deep plantar creases; duplicated collecting system; intestinal malrotation; intrauterine growth retardation; low-set, posteriorly rotated ears; patent ductus arteriosus; prominent nasal tip; pulmonary artery stenosis; sandal gap	/
6	Mendelics, 2019	/	PRKD1	14: 30102151	NM_002742	c.1316G > A	p. Arg439Gln	rs1439477100	Missense	Likely pathogenic	/	/	/	/
7	Shaheen et al., 2015	46XX	PRKD1	14:30093411	NM_002742	c.1852 C > T	p. Arg618Ter	rs201154555	Missense	Pathogenic	Homozygous	CHD	Type I Truncus arteriosus (TA); Cardiomegaly; no other systemic manifestations	25,713,110

No.	Patient	Sex	Gene	Location (GRCh37)	Reference	Nucleotide	Amino acid	SNP ID	Consequence	Pathogenicity/ contribution	Zygosity	CHD classification	Phenotypes	PMID
8	Shaheen et al., 2015	46XX	PRKD1	14:30093411	NM_002742	c.1852 C > T	p. Arg618Ter	rs201154555	Missense	Pathogenic	Homozygous	CHD	Type I truncus arteriosus (TA); Cardiomegaly; no other systemic manifestations	25,713,110
9	Massadeh S, 2021(III-1)	46XX	PRKD1	14:30194881	NM_002742	c.265-1A > G	/	/	Splice acceptor	Pathogenic	Homozygous	CHD	Pulmonary stenosis; normal mental development; normal motor development; normal neurological development	33,919,081
10	Massadeh S, 2021(III-2)	46XX	PRKD1	14:30194881	NM_002742	c.265-1A > G	/	/	Splice acceptor	Pathogenic	Homozygous	CHD	Type II tricuspid regurgitation and, ventricular septal defect (VSD); normal mental development; normal motor development; normal neurological development	33,919,081
11	Massadeh S, 2021(III-3)	46XX	PRKD1	14:30194881	NM_002742	c.265-1A > G	/	/	Splice acceptor	Pathogenic	Homozygous	CHD	Atrial septal defect (ASD); septal defects; normal mental development; normal motor development; normal neurological development	33,919,081
12	Massadeh S, 2021(II-3)	46XX	PRKD1	14:30194881	NM_002742	c.265-1A > G	/	/	Splice acceptor	Pathogenic	Homozygous	CHD	Septal defects; normal mental development; normal motor development; normal neurological development	33,919,081

No.	Patient	Sex	Gene	Location (GRCh37)	Reference	Nucleotide	Amino acid	SNP ID	Consequence	Pathogenicity/ contribution	Zygosity	CHD classification	Phenotypes	PMID
13	Massadeh S, 2021(II-4)	46XX	PRKD1	14:30194881	NM_002742	c.265-1A > G	/	/	Splice acceptor	Pathogenic	Homozygous	CHD	Septal defects; normal mental development; normal motor development; normal neurological development	33,919,081

Table 2.
Clinical information of patients with PRKD1 mutations.

hearing loss, or microcephaly in addition to CHDs [41, 47]. These clinical characteristics bore a striking resemblance to FOXG1-associated encephalopathy. This implied that the haploinsufficiency of PRKD1 might be the causal factor for the syndromic disorder. It is highly probable that PRKD1 and *FOXG1* work together or independently to contribute to the complex clinical manifestations of the congenital variant form of RTT.

According to reports, the serine/threonine protein kinase PRKD1 is involved in several cellular processes, encompassing cell differentiation and migration, the integrity and transport of the Golgi body membrane, the modulation of cell shape and adhesion, and cell survival. It is crucial for synaptic plasticity, synapse development, as well as neuronal polarity [48–50]. These were mediated *via* the MAPK1/3 (ERK1/2) pathway, MAPK8/JNK1, and Ras signaling [51, 52]. In the early stages of oxidative stress, PRKD1 also serves a significant anti-apoptotic survival function for dopaminergic neurons [53]. GWAS indicated that *PRDK1* was linked to intelligence [54], cognitive performance [55], depressive symptoms [56], and susceptibility of Schizophrenia (a psychiatric disorder) [57, 58]. Taken together, *PRKD1* may have a role in the different clinical manifestations of encephalopathies related to FOXG1.

6. Regulatory elements in the intergenic region between *PRKD1* and *FOXG1*

Numerous transcription regulatory elements, including insulators, silencers, and enhancers, are frequently found in intergenic non-coding regions, according to the extensive functional element identifications published by the ENCODE Consortium [59]. Numerous pathogenic CNVs covered all or a portion of the intergenic genomic region between *PRKD1* and *FOXG1* (**Figure 4A-B**). It has been suggested that the pathophysiology of encephalopathy linked to FOXG1 may also include the intergenic *FOXG1-PRKD1*. Remarkably, individuals with encephalopathy related to FOXG1 had five *de novo* inter-chromosomal translocations that eliminated the intergenic *FOXG1-PRKD1* [60, 61]. These translocations removed partial or whole intergenic *FOXG1-PRKD1* and left the promoter and coding sequence of *FOXG1* intact. Therefore, FOXG1 gene is capable of generating proteins with the normal functions.

Regarding the intergenic *FOXG1-PRKD1* area, the majority of CNVs partially or fully overlapped with it (**Figure 4**). This suggests that the *FOXG1-PRKD1* region may have some unidentified roles in FOXG1-related encephalopathies. The human genome (chr14:28,827,675-30,608,124, hg19) was compared with the genomes of other species (chicken, *Xenopus tropicalis*, zebrafish, mouse, rat, opossum, chimpanzee, Rhesus macaque, and dog) by the ECR browser (https://ecrbrowser.dcode.org/). Over evolution, *FOXG1* was highly conserved. Since *PRKD1* was found in mammals, it ought to be regarded as a mammalian-specific gene (**Figure 4D**). In the intergenic *FOXG1-PRKD1* region, eight strongly evolutionary-conserved regions (SECRs) were found (**Figure 4D**). Several regulatory elements may be present in the *FOXG1-PRKD1* area, in accordance with the chromatin modification patterns from the ENCODE study (**Figure 4E**). Additionally, the Open Regulatory Annotation (version 3.0, ORegAnno) database included 14 putative regulatory elements in this genomic area (**Figure 4F**) [62]. SECRs overlapped with most of them. Crucially, using LacZ labeling, 12 potential regulatory elements (70.59%, 12/14) were examined for enhancer activity in mouse embryos (E11.5) [63]. Six SECRs functioned as active enhancers: two in the hindbrain (hs1168 and hs1539), one in the neural tube (hs598), and three in the mouse forebrain (hs342, hs1523, and hs566) (**Figure 4G-H**). This indicated that these

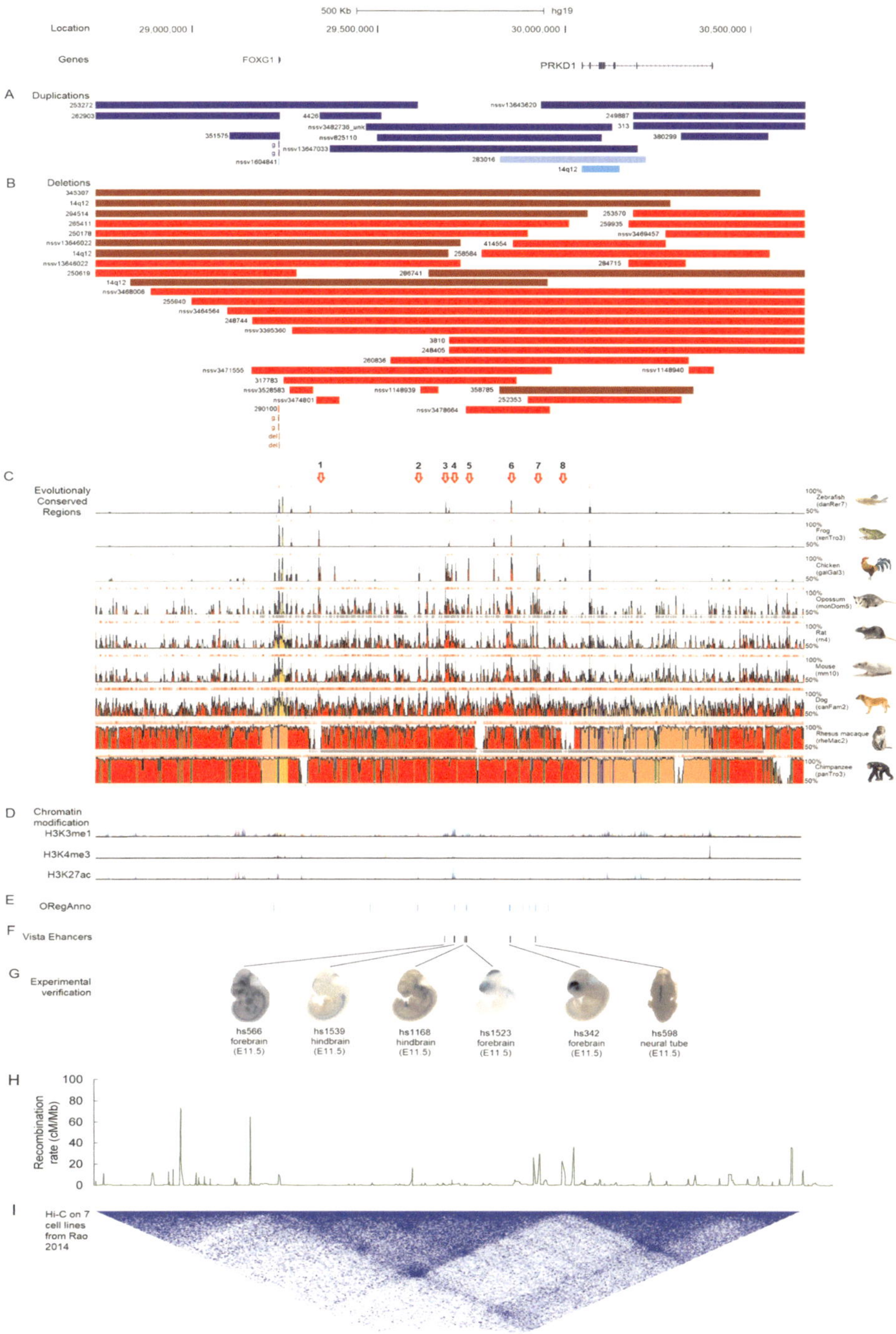

Figure 4.
Characteristic analysis of regulatory elements in the intergenic region between PRKD1 and FOXG1. (A) Partially covered microduplications; (B) microdeletions; (C) chromosomal translocations; (D) evolutional conservation analysis via *the ECR browser; (E) chromatin modifications in seven human cell types from ENCODE; (F) regulatory elements in ORegAnno database; (G) enhancers in VISTA enhancer browser; (H) six neuroactive enhancers in mouse embryos; (I)* in situ *Hi-C for seven human cell lines (Adopted from Lu et al. [2]).*

enhancers might be functioned specifically in neurons. Since enhancers could function long-distantly and bi-directionally.

This intergenic *FOXG1-PRKD1* region comprises three topologically-associating domains (TADs), according to an analysis of *in situ* Hi-C (High-through Chromosome Conformation Capture) data for seven human cell lines (KBM7, K562, GM12878, HUVEC, HMEC, NHEK, and IMR90) (GEO: GSE63525) [64]. The second TADs contained both *FOXG1* and the intergenic region (*FOXG1-PRKD1*) (**Figure 4I**). The last enhancer (element_555), 760 kb downstream of *FOXG1*, was located in close vicinity to a schizophrenia-related SNP (rs1191551) in this TAD. According to the Luciferase reporter experiment, the short area containing rs1191551 was able to modulate *FOXG1* expression but not *PRKD1* [65, 66]. FOXG1 expression was considerably reduced after CRISR-Cas9 removed the region containing rs1191551, whereas PRKD1 expression remained unaffected [65, 66]. This supports the idea that the pathogenic chromosomal rearrangements or microdeletions involving the intergenic *FOXG1-PRKD1* result in FOXG1-related disorders by disrupting the regulatory activities of distant regulatory enhancers on FOXG1 expression.

Furthermore, according to the significant single-tissue eQTLs data for *PRKD1* and *FOXG1* in GTEx database, 137 eQTLs were found only in the FOXG1-specific TAD. For the 214 eQTLs linked to *PRKD1* expression, only two (rs78802132 and rs80019464, 0.93%) were found in the FOXG1-specific TAD (**Figure 5A**). These results indicate that, under the cis-acting model, intergenic regulatory elements primarily modulate the expression of *FOXG1* rather than *PRKD1*. Nevertheless, numerous transcription factors regulate FOXG1 expression, and the regulatory mechanisms of intergenic enhancers remain unclear. This indicated that the haploinsufficiency of

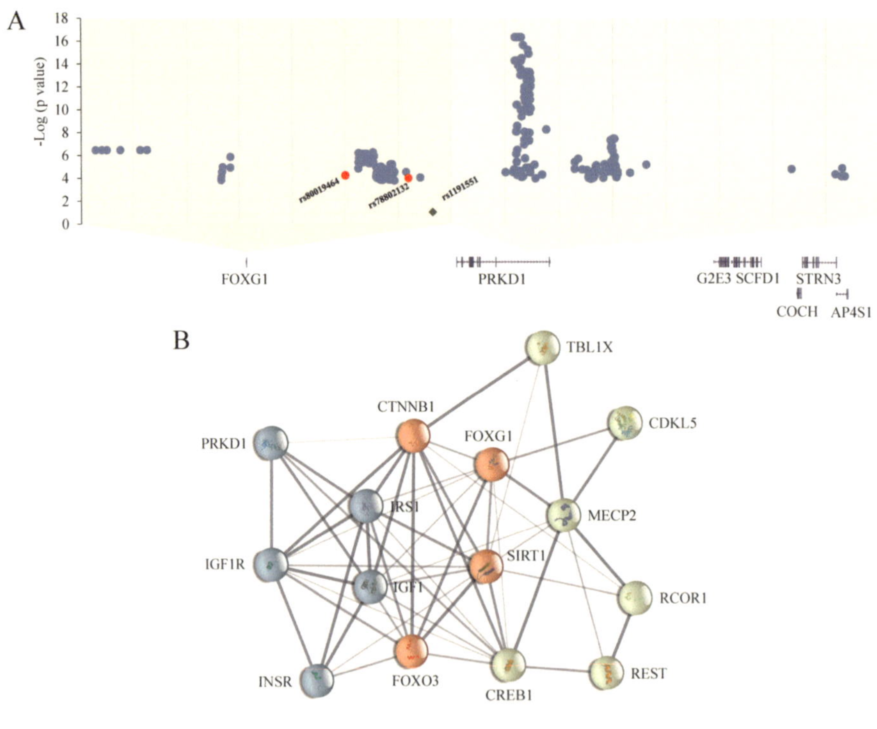

Figure 5.
eQTLs and STRINGed network analysis for PRKD1 and FOXG1. (A) eQTLs for PRKD1 and FOXG1; (B) STRINGed protein interaction network (Adopted from Lu et al. [2]).

FOXG1 could be caused by several mechanisms, (1) frameshifting mutations; (2) nonsense mutations; (3) microdeletions of FOXG1; and (4) microdeletions of non-coding intergenic region of *FOXG1-PRKD1.*

7. The relationship between FOXG1 and PRKD1

It has been reported that IGF-1/IGF-1R pathway could recruit and activate MAPK/ERK and PI3K/mTOR pathways to regulate cell cycle/survival, gene expression, and cytoskeleton remodeling, which were important for neuronal development. Functional recovery with the recombinant human IGF1 has been investigated as a therapy option in mouse models of Rett syndrome [67–69] and a patient with Rett syndrome [70], both achieved exciting results. In order to infer the relationship of these genes, a STRING analysis was performed for reported RTT-like or RTT genes, for instance, FOXG1, CDKL5 and MECP2, plus IGF1, PRKD1, INSR, and IGF1R (**Figure 5B**). FOXG1 may interact with CDKL5 and MECP2. The INSR-IRS1 complex and the IGF1-IGF1R complex may directly control FOXG1 expression while indirectly controlling CKDL5 and MECP2 expression. Regarding PRKD1, it has been documented that it may interact with IGF1R [71]. It suggested that the pathogenesis of RTT-like or RTT syndrome may be considerably influenced by insulin or the insulin-like factor pathway. IGF1 may enhance some clinical manifestations in clinical trials and RTT-relevant phenotypes in animal models [68–72]. Given its capacity to bind or control IGF1R expression, PRKD1 is most likely a novel, significant causative or contributing element to the clinical manifestations of encephalopathy related to FOXG1. To determine the effect of PRKD1 in the pathogenesis of encephalopathy related to FOXG1, experiments under the animal and cellular levels should be conducted.

8. Conclusions

Our thorough reanalysis of FOXG1 mutations reveals that the molecular pathogenesis of FOXG1-associated disorders was highly complex. This may be induced by mutations within the CDS of FOXG1 itself, microduplication or microdeletion of the whole FOXG1 and the regulatory elements in the intergenic *FOXG1-PRKD1* region, as well as PRKD1 modification. For medical professionals, the treatment of FOXG1-related encephalopathy is extremely difficult.

Author contributions

G.L and Q.P conceived the project and drafted and revised the manuscript. G.L. conducted clinical data analysis and genetic counseling. G.M and Q.P conducted the data analysis and bibliographic search. G.M and Q.P collected data and recruited mutations. Q.P was the corresponding author. All authors critically revised the important academic content of this paper.

Funding

This research was financially supported by Key Research and Development Project of Deyang Science and Technology Bureau (2024SZY004), Special Fund for

Incubation Projects of Deyang People's Hospital (FHR202501, FHR202502), and Natural Science Foundation of Sichuan Province (2022NSFSC0714).

Competing interests

There are no conflicts of interest between authors or funding sources.

Ethics approval statement

This study was performed following the Code of Ethics of the World Medical Association (Declaration of Helsinki), which applies to experiments involving human subjects. This study has been authorized by the Ethical Committee of the Shenzhen Baoan Women's and Children's Hospital. All of the participants in the research gave their written informed consent. The parents or legal guardians of the minors provided written informed consent.

Author details

Guanting Lu[1,2], Gang Mai[3] and Qiongling Peng[4]*

1 Laboratory of Translational Medicine Research, Department of Pathology, Deyang People's Hospital, Jingyang District, Deyang, China

2 Key Laboratory of Tumor Molecular Research of Deyang, Jingyang District, Deyang, China

3 Center of Hepatopancreatobiliary Surgery, Deyang People's Hospital, Jingyang District, Deyang, China

4 Department of Child Healthcare, Shenzhen Baoan Women's and Children's Hospital, Shenzhen University, Baoan District, Shenzhen, China

*Address all correspondence to: pql1016@126.com

References

[1] Grillo E et al. Rett networked database: An integrated clinical and genetic network of Rett syndrome databases. Human Mutation. 2012;**33**(7): 1031-1036

[2] Lu G et al. Identification of a de novo mutation of the FOXG1 gene and comprehensive analysis for molecular factors in Chinese FOXG1-related encephalopathies. Frontiers in Molecular Neuroscience. 2022;**15**:1039990

[3] Moog U et al. Neurodevelopmental disorders in males related to the gene causing Rett syndrome in females (MECP2). European Journal of Paediatric Neurology. 2003;**7**(1):5-12

[4] Byun CK et al. FOXG1 mutation is a low-incidence genetic cause in atypical Rett syndrome. Child Neurology Open. 2015;**2**(1):2329048X14568151

[5] Brimble E et al. Expanding genotype-phenotype correlations in FOXG1 syndrome: Results from a patient registry. Orphanet Journal of Rare Diseases. 2023;**18**(1):149

[6] Mitter D et al. FOXG1 syndrome: Genotype-phenotype association in 83 patients with FOXG1 variants. Genetics in Medicine. 2018;**20**(1):98-108

[7] Wong LC et al. FOXG1-related syndrome: From clinical to molecular genetics and pathogenic mechanisms. International Journal of Molecular Sciences. 2019;**20**(17):4176

[8] McMahon KQ et al. Familial recurrences of FOXG1-related disorder: Evidence for mosaicism. American Journal of Medical Genetics. Part A. 2015;**167A**(12):3096-3102

[9] Wong LC et al. Cognition and evolution of movement disorders of FOXG1-related syndrome. Frontiers in Neurology. 2019;**10**:641

[10] Toresson H et al. Conservation of BF-1 expression in amphioxus and zebrafish suggests evolutionary ancestry of anterior cell types that contribute to the vertebrate telencephalon. Development Genes and Evolution. 1998;**208**(8):431-439

[11] Manuel M et al. The transcription factor Foxg1 regulates the competence of telencephalic cells to adopt subpallial fates in mice. Development. 2010;**137**(3): 487-497

[12] Miyoshi G et al. FoxG1 regulates the formation of cortical GABAergic circuit during an early postnatal critical period resulting in autism spectrum disorder-like phenotypes. Nature Communications. 2021;**12**(1):1-17

[13] Chiola S et al. Foxg1 overexpression in neocortical pyramids stimulates dendrite elongation via Hes1 and pCreb1 upregulation. Cerebral Cortex. 2019;**29**(3):1006-1019

[14] Dastidar SG, Landrieu PMZ, D'Mello SR. FoxG1 promotes the survival of postmitotic neurons. Journal of Neuroscience. 2011;**31**(2):402-413

[15] Yu B et al. Disruption of Foxg1 impairs neural plasticity leading to social and cognitive behavioral defects. Molecular Brain. 2019;**12**(1):1-12

[16] Tian C et al. Foxg1 has an essential role in postnatal development of the dentate gyrus. Journal of Neuroscience. 2012;**32**(9):2931-2949

[17] Pande S et al. De novo variants underlying monogenic syndromes with intellectual disability in a

neurodevelopmental cohort from India. European Journal of Human Genetics. 2024;**32**(10):1291-1298

[18] Ghasemi MR et al. Exome sequencing reveals neurodevelopmental genes in simplex consanguineous Iranian families with syndromic autism. BMC Medical Genomics. 2024;**17**(1):196

[19] Lin TY et al. Functional defects in FOXG1 variants predict the severity of brain anomalies in FOXG1 syndrome. Molecular Psychiatry. 2025;**30**(10):4824-4835

[20] Hu Q et al. A novel frameshift mutation of FOXG1-induced congenital variant of Rett syndrome: A case report. Asian Journal of Surgery. 2024;**47**(7): 3211-3213

[21] Zhang Q et al. Novel FOXG1 mutations in Chinese patients with Rett syndrome or Rett-like mental retardation. BMC Medical Genetics. 2017;**18**(1):1-6

[22] Niu Y et al. A case of congenital Rett variant in a Chinese patient caused by a FOXG1 mutation. Annals of Saudi Medicine. 2020;**40**(4):347-353

[23] Bai Y et al. Genotype-phenotype implications from three representative clinical FOXG1 variants associated with FOXG1 syndrome. Seizure. 2021;**89**:45-47

[24] Li S, Sun G, Zhao G, Kong X. Analysis of a case with heterozygous 14q12 deletion and FOXG1 gene-related disease. Zhonghua Yi Xue Yi Chuan Xue Za Zhi. 2021;**38**(4):366-368

[25] Tang Z, Tong G, Hong L, Zhou T, Xu Y. Application value of chromosome microarray analysis in the genetic etiology of children with unexplained intellectual disability/developmental delay. Journal of Anhui Health Vocational & Technical College. 2021; **20**:121-124

[26] Wang F et al. Report of a case with 14q12 triplication and literature review for FOXG1 related diseases. Zhonghua yi xue yi chuan xue za zhi= Zhonghua yixue yichuanxue zazhi=Chinese Journal of Medical Genetics. 2017;**34**(5):671-675

[27] Cui L, Yue L, Chen L, Jia R, Zhaoxuan W, Tan X, et al. A case of Congenital Rett syndrome variant caused by FOXG1 gene mutation. Chinese Medical Case Repository. 2023; **5**:e00048

[28] Sun D, Wang Y, Li J, Zhang L, Hou M. Analysis of clinical and genetic detection results of 3 children with FOXG1-related syndrome. Journal of Clinical Pediatrics. 2024;**42**(9):805-810

[29] Richards S et al. Standards and guidelines for the interpretation of sequence variants: A joint consensus recommendation of the American College of Medical Genetics and Genomics and the Association for Molecular Pathology. Genetics in Medicine. 2015;**17**(5):405-423

[30] Vegas N et al. Delineating FOXG1 syndrome: From congenital microcephaly to hyperkinetic encephalopathy. Neurology Genetics. 2018;**4**(6):e281

[31] Nykamp K et al. Sherloc: A comprehensive refinement of the ACMG–AMP variant classification criteria. Genetics in Medicine. 2017;**19** (10):1105-1117

[32] Cellini E et al. The hyperkinetic movement disorder of FOXG 1-related epileptic–dyskinetic encephalopathy. Developmental Medicine and Child Neurology. 2016;**58**(1):93-97

[33] Seltzer LE et al. Epilepsy and outcome in FOXG1-related disorders. Epilepsia. 2014;**55**(8):1292-1300

[34] Bean LJ et al. Free the data: One laboratory's approach to knowledge-based genomic variant classification and preparation for EMR integration of genomic data. Human Mutation. 2013;**34**(9):1183-1188

[35] Van der Aa N et al. Analysis of FOXG1 is highly recommended in male and female patients with Rett syndrome. Molecular Syndromology. 2010;**1**(6):290-293

[36] Kortüm F et al. The core FOXG1 syndrome phenotype consists of postnatal microcephaly, severe mental retardation, absent language, dyskinesia, and corpus callosum hypogenesis. Journal of Medical Genetics. 2011;**48**(6):396-406

[37] Bahi-Buisson N et al. Revisiting the phenotype associated with FOXG1 mutations: Two novel cases of congenital Rett variant. Neurogenetics. 2010;**11**(2):241-249

[38] Kurosaki T, Popp MW, Maquat LE. Quality and quantity control of gene expression by nonsense-mediated mRNA decay. Nature Reviews. Molecular Cell Biology. 2019;**20**(7):406-420

[39] Cooper GM et al. A copy number variation morbidity map of developmental delay. Nature Genetics. 2011;**43**(9):838-846

[40] Coe BP et al. Refining analyses of copy number variation identifies specific genes associated with developmental delay. Nature Genetics. 2014;**46**(10):1063-1071

[41] Sifrim A et al. Distinct genetic architectures for syndromic and nonsyndromic congenital heart defects identified by exome sequencing. Nature Genetics. 2016;**48**(9):1060-1065

[42] Massadeh S et al. Novel autosomal recessive splice-altering variant in PRKD1 is associated with congenital heart disease. Genes. 2021;**12**(5):612

[43] Shaheen R et al. Positional mapping of PRKD1, NRP1 and PRDM1 as novel candidate disease genes in truncus arteriosus. Journal of Medical Genetics. 2015;**52**(5):322-329

[44] Monies D et al. Lessons learned from large-scale, first-tier clinical exome sequencing in a highly consanguineous population. American Journal of Human Genetics. 2019;**6**:1182-1201

[45] Qazi Waheed-Ullah AW, Abbad A, Rochette S, Bu'Lock F, Hitz M-P, Dombrowsky G, et al. Effect of deletion of the protein kinase PRKD1 on development of the mouse embryonic heart. Journal of Anatomy. 2024;**1**:1

[46] Watanabe D et al. Brain calcification in congenital heart defects and ectodermal dysplasia (CHDED). European Journal of Medical Genetics. 2025;**73**:104992

[47] Swaminathan GJ et al. DECIPHER: Web-based, community resource for clinical interpretation of rare variants in developmental disorders. Human Molecular Genetics. 2012;**21**(R1):R37-R44

[48] Bisbal M et al. Protein kinase d regulates trafficking of dendritic membrane proteins in developing neurons. Journal of Neuroscience. 2008;**28**(37):9297-9308

[49] Yin D-M et al. Both the establishment and maintenance of neuronal polarity require the activity of protein kinase D in the Golgi apparatus.

Journal of Neuroscience. 2008;**28**(35):8832-8843

[50] Cen C et al. PKD1 promotes functional synapse formation coordinated with N-cadherin in hippocampus. Journal of Neuroscience. 2018;**38**(1):183-199

[51] Hao F et al. LPA(1)-mediated PKD2 activation promotes LPA-induced tissue factor expression via the p38alpha and JNK2 MAPK pathways in smooth muscle cells. The Journal of Biological Chemistry. 2021;**297**(4):101152

[52] Wang P et al. Protein kinase D1 is essential for Ras-induced senescence and tumor suppression by regulating senescence-associated inflammation. Proceedings of the National Academy of Sciences of the United States of America. 2014;**111**(21):7683-7688

[53] Asaithambi A et al. Protein kinase D1 (PKD1) activation mediates a compensatory protective response during early stages of oxidative stress-induced neuronal degeneration. Molecular Neurodegeneration. 2011;**6**(1):1-19

[54] Hill WD et al. A combined analysis of genetically correlated traits identifies 187 loci and a role for neurogenesis and myelination in intelligence. Molecular Psychiatry. 2019;**24**(2):169-181

[55] Lee JJ et al. Gene discovery and polygenic prediction from a genome-wide association study of educational attainment in 1.1 million individuals. Nature Genetics. 2018;**50**(8):1112-1121

[56] Baselmans BM et al. Multivariate genome-wide analyses of the well-being spectrum. Nature Genetics. 2019;**51**(3):445-451

[57] Ripke S et al. Biological insights from 108 schizophrenia-associated genetic loci. Nature. 2014;**511**(7510):421

[58] Wu Y et al. Multi-trait analysis for genome-wide association study of five psychiatric disorders. Translational Psychiatry. 2020;**10**(1):1-11

[59] Maurano MT et al. Systematic localization of common disease-associated variation in regulatory DNA. Science. 2012;**337**(6099):1190-1195

[60] Goubau C et al. Platelet defects in congenital variant of Rett syndrome patients with FOXG1 mutations or reduced expression due to a position effect at 14q12. European Journal of Human Genetics. 2013;**21**(12):1349-1355

[61] Mehrjouy MM et al. Regulatory variants of FOXG1 in the context of its topological domain organisation. European Journal of Human Genetics. 2018;**26**(2):186-196

[62] Lesurf R et al. ORegAnno 3.0: A community-driven resource for curated regulatory annotation. Nucleic Acids Research. 2016;**44**(D1):D126-D132

[63] Visel A et al. VISTA enhancer browser—A database of tissue-specific human enhancers. Nucleic Acids Research. 2007;**35**(suppl_1):D88-D92

[64] Rao SS et al. A 3D map of the human genome at kilobase resolution reveals principles of chromatin looping. Cell. 2014;**159**(7):1665-1680

[65] Won H et al. Chromosome conformation elucidates regulatory relationships in developing human brain. Nature. 2016;**538**(7626):523-527

[66] Hamerlinck L et al. Non-coding structural variants identify a commonly affected regulatory region steering FOXG1 transcription in early neurodevelopment. medRxiv. 2025:2025.03.10.25323301. DOI: 10.1101/2025.03.10.25323301

[67] Gigliucci V et al. Region-specific KCC2 rescue by rhIGF-1 and oxytocin in a mouse model of Rett syndrome. Cerebral Cortex. 2022;**32**(13):2885-2894

[68] Keogh C et al. Functional network mapping reveals state-dependent response to IGF1 treatment in Rett syndrome. Brain Sciences. 2020;**10**(8): 515

[69] Bray N. Neurodevelopmental disorders: Righting Rett syndrome with IGF1. Nature Reviews. Drug Discovery. 2014;**13**(9):653

[70] Pini G et al. Repeated insulin-like growth factor 1 treatment in a patient with rett syndrome: A single case study. Frontiers in Pediatrics. 2014;**2**:52

[71] Hermanto U et al. RACK1, an insulin-like growth factor I (IGF-I) receptor-interacting protein, modulates IGF-I-dependent integrin signaling and promotes cell spreading and contact with extracellular matrix. Molecular and Cellular Biology. 2002;**22**(7):2345-2365

[72] Pini G et al. IGF1 as a potential treatment for Rett syndrome: Safety assessment in six Rett patients. Autism Research and Treatment. 2012;**2012**: 679801

Chapter 5

Perspective Chapter: From Embryonic Archives to Translational Insights – Reusing Nonhuman Primate Brain Data to Decode Development and Reduce Animal Sacrifice

Alvaro Duque, Phil Barello, Lucy Greene, Emma Burke, Valeria Mendoza-Silva, Yury M. Morozov and Pasko Rakic

Abstract

A serious challenge when conducting studies of neurogenesis and brain development in nonhuman primates (NHPs) is the lack of sufficient, homogeneous data and methodologies to assure accurate, repeatable studies. Matching of age, sex, histological processes, and planes of orientation is paramount, and hence, standards need to be set as a basis for comparisons between normal controls and specimens with lesions, treatments, or pathologies. Part of the challenge is that during development, everything is rapidly changing. Even a few days' mismatch in embryonic age can translate into sizable differences in structural maturity in some brain areas. Sexual dimorphism in the embryonic rhesus macaque is evidenced by differences in average body and brain size and weight at birth. Hence, comparisons of cortical and subcortical regions, glia, neurons, and axonal pathways necessitate the normalization of data with enough matching specimens to ensure meaningful and accurate averages. Natural interindividual variability plays a role and increases the statistical variance in otherwise identical samples. As a solution to this problem, we propose an increase in the sharing and archiving of specimens and data, which ultimately results in an increase in the number of available samples for analysis. This is achievable by building well-documented, accurate, and reliable embryonic datasets. This chapter introduces the creation of such datasets within Collection 6 of the MacBrain Resource Center (MBRC) as a standard for assuring transparency, accuracy, reliability, and repeatability of developmental NHP brain studies. This effort is based on the extended use of materials collected from unrelated studies.

Keywords: rhesus macaque, embryo, MacBrain Resource Center, study reproducibility, decreased animal use, 3Rs

1. Introduction

Most studies of brain development using macaques are rather limited in terms of the number of animals and the completeness of samples per age, sex, and histological repertoire. Repeated imaging of the fetal brain by ultrasound or MRI usually requires repeated anesthesia of the mother, which introduces anesthetic agents, stress, and anxiety as confounding factors. These methods may be globally informative but insufficient. Repeated imaging may, therefore, be impractical and may, in addition, not provide sufficient cytoarchitectonic resolution. Histological processing of one sample is not repeatable in the same specimen at different ages, but it is unsurpassed in terms of cyto-resolution. Obviously, C-sections are required for the collection of the specimens, and if a particular sex is desirable, a priori determination of the sex is also needed. In any case, accurate embryonic age is challenging because it requires precision in the timing of pregnancy and very accurate measurement of crown-rump lengths as a proxy for age if imaging is being used to estimate it. Once an embryo is collected, brain tissue processing is not precisely easy because the samples are usually very fragile, and if fixation is limited to immersion, a proper balance between fixation strength, exposure time, and quality histo- and immunohistochemistry needs to be achieved. The production of embryos requires a breeding colony, and the collection of embryos requires experienced and specialized veterinary medical personnel able to perform C-sections and subsequently care for the recovery of the mother.

Given the difficulties in procuring NHP embryos for studies of brain development, the building of accurate and reliable datasets with reusable information seems not only justifiable but necessary to foster and facilitate developmental brain research. The building of such a database is challenging and expensive, but it is underway within the MacBrain Resource Center (MBRC) in the Department of Neuroscience at the Yale University School of Medicine. Making all data publicly available constitutes true data sharing that encourages data reuse, promotes discovery, enhances scientific rigor, and diminishes costs, both in terms of animal lives and in terms of the financial burden of data production. Some fundamental aspects of scientific importance are the proper documentation of data collection and characterization and the proper and safe storage of the data while still assuring a user-friendly interface. These aspects are crucial for data reuse and repeated analysis using ever-changing analytical tools.

Here, we describe our efforts to provide the scientific community with such a database. As rhesus macaque embryos have been collected for unrelated studies, we get what is left over and not needed by those original studies, and process available brain tissue further in an organized and systematic way. Our data repository is intended to be the already established and operational Collection 6 of the MBRC (https://macbraingallery.yale.edu/collection6/). For completeness, the descriptions below cover from specimen procurement to examples of data analysis.

2. Procurement of the specimens

2.1 The breeding colony: Production of timed pregnancies

The production of timed pregnancies is a process that starts with daily vaginal swabs. In time, the females get accustomed to the process, and with the help of positive reinforcement, they readily present. The collection is done with the tip of a cotton applicator for the detection of menstrual blood, which is subsequently used to estimate the time of ovulation. The female in heat is paired with the male for ~72 hours, that is, for three nights, starting around the morning of the 10th day after the onset of menstruation. The male and female are separated on the morning of the 4th day. During this time, the pair usually copulates several times. In the case of a proven pregnancy, the approximate time of conception is estimated to be the middle of the second day of pairing, so our uncertainty is ~ ±1.5 days. This can, of course, be longer given the possible long survival of the sperm before the fertilization of the egg. The estimate has, however, over the years, proved to be accurate enough for our purposes.

2.2 The determination of sex

When necessary, the determination of embryo sex is done by testing maternal blood serum for the presence of the DNA sex-determining region of the Y gene (SRY). This is done in-house by polymerase chain reaction (PCR) following the protocol described by Mitsunaga et al., [1]. To increase accuracy, blood from the pregnant macaque is preferably obtained ~35 days or later after pairing.

2.3 Collection of embryos

C-sections are performed by qualified veterinarians at the embryonic age specified by research needs (see **Figure 1**). A team of experts performs the surgeries following the same high medical standards followed in the human procedure. There is always a dedicated surgeon and a dedicated anesthesiologist. Several veterinary medical assistants help monitor vital signs and handle surgical instruments. Pre- and postoperative care is also managed by professionals, which always include veterinary residents who conduct daily clinical rounds. The husbandry staff is highly qualified to recognize and report any signs of distress. After euthanasia by sodium pentobarbital overdose, larger embryos are usually transcardially perfused with 0.1 M phosphate buffer saline (PBS), followed by 4% paraformaldehyde (PF) and 15% picric acid in PBS (Zamboni fixative). In the case of smaller embryos, the whole head or even the whole body may be fixed by immersion in the same fixative. In these cases, the fontanelle is usually opened with the tip of a surgical blade to aid the fixative solution in reaching the brain. Immersion is usually overnight, and the same is done for older brains, but postfixation may be longer depending on the quality of the primary fixation. Cryoprotection is done in 20–30% sucrose in PBS for as long as needed until the brain sinks in the solution. Timing depends on the size of the brain, which is a function of age.

2.4 Brain cutting and tissue storage

After proper cryoprotection, brains are either blocked or stored whole. They are frozen in isopentane surrounded by dry ice and stored at −80°C. To produce different series of sections that can be systematically processed for different histological markers, we prefer to cut sections at 50 microns thick in a cryostat (Leica CM1950) (See **Figure 2**). Most of the tissue is cut in the coronal plane, but there are instances in which it is cut in sagittal or axial orientations. When a complete brain or a complete hemisphere is available, we cut the whole rostral-to-caudal extent, and depending on the size and number of sections that are acquired (which depends on brain size determined by age), we select a set number of series to be processed so that each series is processed for a single marker, and the sections within each series are equidistant. For instance, from a 15 mm brain, we obtain 300 coronal sections. In a case like

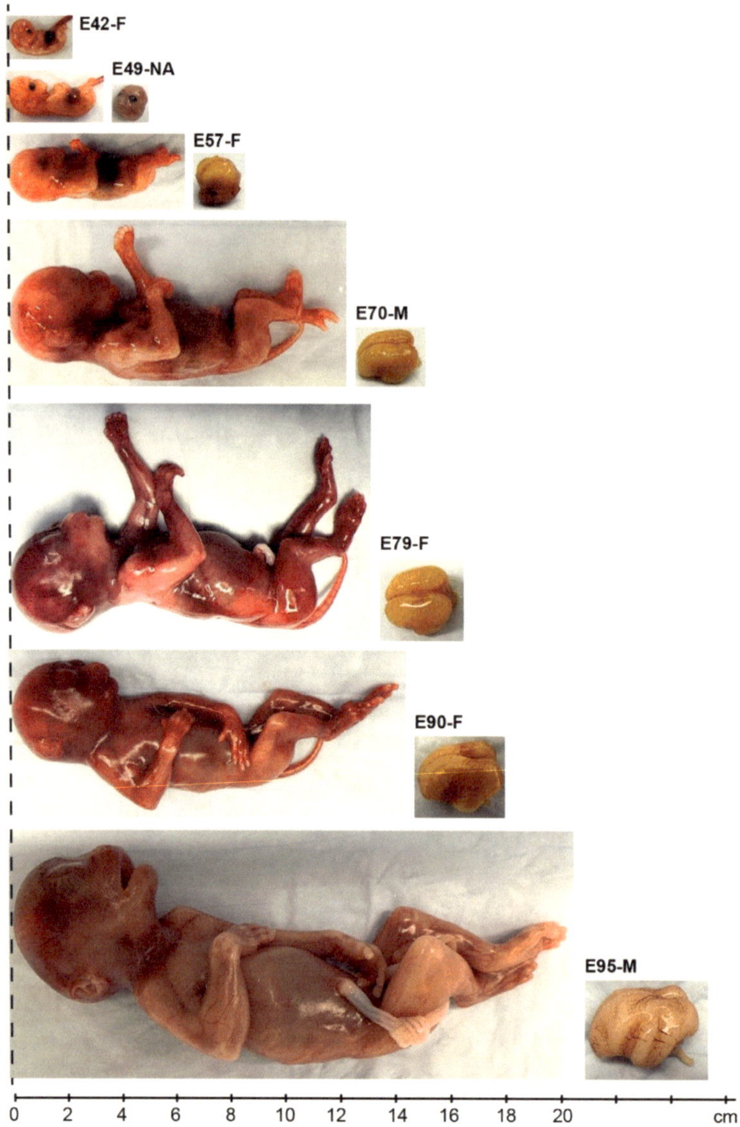

Figure 1.
Examples of rhesus macaque embryos of different ages and sexes. Seven specimens are arranged top to bottom by age ± 1.5 days. Images of the head or brain are also provided from E49 to E95; all images are to scale. The large variability of body sizes is easily appreciated and helps understand the need to collect several specimens of the same sex and age in order to obtain averaged data more truly representative of the population. Abbreviations: male (M), female (F), not available (NA).

this, one can separate 10 series of 30 sections each. For younger embryos with smaller brains, it may be necessary to collect more specimens, since the number of different labels that can be done in one brain is limited by brain size. Sections that are too far apart may fail to properly sample a small developing structure. Too many sections per series decrease the number of different series that can be obtained per specimen. We try to balance the sampling rates to maximize the amount of information that can be obtained per specimen while, at the same time, trying to decrease the number of specimens that are needed. Since the specimens that make it to the MBRC collections

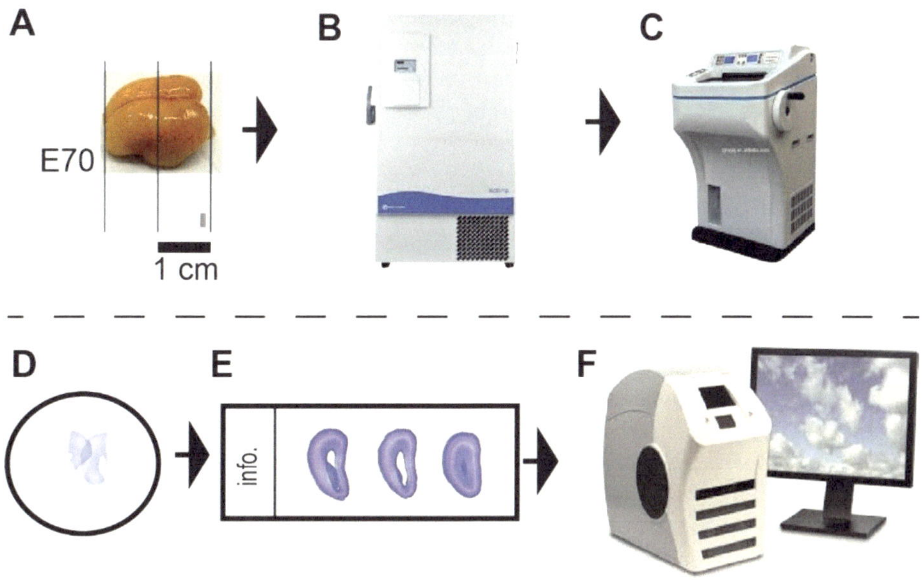

Figure 2.
Storing, cutting, staining, glass mounting, and digitization of brain sections. Fixed and cryoprotected brains (A) are stored at −80°C (B) until cut in a cryostat (C). Sections were then processed free-floating (if possible) (D) and mounted on glass slides (E). After further processing and cover slipping, they are digitized (F).

are left over from unrelated experiments, it may be the case that only one hemisphere is available or that just a few blocks of tissue are available; whatever the case, we try to maximize the amount of tissue that can be processed in an effort to, in time, decrease the need to sacrifice additional animals.

2.5 Histo- and immunohistochemistry processing

Over the years, our histological processes have been described in detail in different publications [2–12]. All histological processing is done free-floating unless it is not possible, such as may be the case with the youngest specimens, in which case they are processed on the slide. All solutions are prepared in PBS. Sections are always rinsed 2x or 3x in PBS and endogenous peroxidases inactivated with 0.2–0.5% H_2O_2 for about 2 and to 20 minutes. After further rinsing, sections are incubated in solutions containing the primary antibody for 24–36 hours at room temperature (RT). Proper dilutions are empirically predetermined and vary from antibody to antibody. Typical dilutions are 1:1000 to 1:10,000. Oftentimes, the solution with the primary antibody also contains 0.2% Triton X to improve antibody penetration. After rinsing, sections are incubated in appropriate biotinylated secondary antibodies. Typical dilutions are 1:200 to 1:500, and the solution typically contains 2–5% serum from the host of the secondary antibody and may also have the same concentration of bovine serum albumin (BSA). All these steps are intended to decrease nonspecific background staining, resulting in a better signal-to-noise ratio. Incubation is usually at RT for 4–8 hours. After rinsing, a final incubation is done in avidin-biotin-peroxidase complex (Vectastain elite ABC kit, Vector labs, Burlingame, CA) for 4 hours at RT, following the manufacturer's recommended dilution. The development of the immunoreaction product is done with 3′,3′-diaminobenzidine as chromogen precipitated by H_2O_2 [10, 12–14]. After washing, the sections are mounted on microscope glass slides, dried, dehydrated in a series of alcohols, cleared in xylenes, and cover-slipped with Permount® (Fisher Scientific, Fair Lawn, NJ). In general, embryonic tissue is much more delicate than adult tissue. It has less neuropil and a higher water content. Adjustments are usually necessary on a case-by-case basis to preserve tissue integrity and improve quality.

2.6 Imaging and digitization of sections and digital data storage

The MBRC performs ScanScope Virtual Slide (SVS, slide and viewable storage) image file ingest using the Aperio CS2 image capture device, driven by Aperio ScanScope software, to store digitized microscope slides at up to 40x magnification. Physical microscope slides are digitally scanned, and the SVS image files are organized in a database, stored in our network-accessible storage repository, and accessible in an Aperio eSlideManager web interface that includes a full-resolution viewer capable of displaying whole-slide images through a web browser to authenticated visitors. Alternatively, Aperio ImageScope software is an option limited to devices running a Microsoft Windows operating system. A monthly fee is incurred based on the amount of data stored. University information technology support (ITS) experts oversee data integrity and security. If necessary, slides can also be scanned by a different scanner, such as the Zeiss Axioscan 7, an Olympus VS200, or a Huron TissueScope.

2.7 Construction of public web galleries of whole-slide images

Because the Aperio CS2 HR scanner has been our primary instrument in the digitization of data, the descriptions that follow are targeted to this system. However, the principles are the same, independent of the system employed.

2.7.1 Digital input

Aperio ScanScope Virtual Slide (SVS) images are big-tagged image file format (TIFF) files "fully compatible with the TIFF standard, with no proprietary extensions" [15]. Whereas the original TIFF image standard allowed for a maximum file size of 4 GB, BigTIFF images use 64-bit offsets, supporting image sizes up to 18 exabytes (EB).

SVS images include image details, with slide image data stored using lossy JPEG2000 compression and a macro view in low resolution of the slide label stored with lossless Lempel–Ziv–Welch (LZW) compression. The first image in the set of images contained within an SVS file is always a full-resolution tiled baseline image, usually 240 × 240 pixels [15], and the second image is a 1024 × 768-pixel stripped thumbnail of the macro, followed by a set of one or more intermediate pyramidal images, which are compressed with the same algorithm as the base image, and an optional final slide label image.

Leica Biosystems maintains Aperio eSlideManager, which was previously developed by Aperio Technologies, Inc. Aperio eSlideManager is a digital pathology system of record.

2.7.2 Conversion process

Individual SVS image files can be located within the storage repository using the ImageID value displayed within the eSlideManager web interface, originally assigned by the eSlideManager database. To make Aperio SVS images more accessible, without requiring visitors to install software plugins or provide login credentials, the MBRC leveraged OpenSlide, a software interface to whole-slide images in multiple image formats, including SVS [16]. Deep Zoom image format is XML-based and supports single images, sparse images with multiple regions having different dimensions, and collections of multiple images [17]. Each Deep Zoom image is stored as a tiled pyramid with a 2-dimensional (height and width) base. Every level of the pyramid, from the tip of the peak with the fewest pixels at level 0 to the lowest level, which varies by image height and width values, is a 256-tile image.

Each Aperio SVS image file can be converted to Deep Zoom image format using libvips, an open-source image processing library compatible with OpenSlide image files. OpenSlide enables libvips to operate as a bridge between the Aperio SVS image format and Deep Zoom and other International Image Interoperability Framework (IIIF) image formats.

Creating a single Deep Zoom image from an SVS image requires a computer with sufficient software and hardware. When creating multiple Deep Zoom images in parallel on one computer, working memory and local storage can become overloaded, and image conversion will not proceed without intervention. To limit the overloading of the working memory or local storage of the virtual servers for image conversion, the MBRC implemented a distributed computing approach. To create a web gallery of multiple SVS images, each SVS image file is sent to one of several virtual servers in a fleet that allows for server rotation, expansion, and gradual replacement. Three virtual servers operating in parallel can convert 100 SVS image files, distributed as a subset of complete individual SVS images, to Deep Zoom images within a few hours. It is possible to expand this fleet to include many more virtual servers that can accept SVS image files as input, convert the SVS images to Deep Zoom images with libvips, and deliver the Deep Zoom image files to long-term storage. For example, for a gallery with 100 brain sections (i.e., 100 SVS images), 70 images can be converted by the first and third servers (35 each), and 30 by the second server, assuming they are handling sections in rostral-to-caudal order. The reason for the uneven number distribution is that approximately the first 20 rostral images and the last 20 caudal images of a whole brain sliced coronally are generally smaller files based on the physical size of the brain at the rostral and caudal extremes. The intermediate sections are physically larger, represented by logically larger image files, which justifies a variable distribution of work among the servers.

In summary, each SVS image file is located within the eSlideManager storage repository and copied to local storage on the virtual server. SVS image file conversion to Deep Zoom format is performed on local storage. SVS images are distributed in parallel to one of a fleet of virtual servers with libvips and access to the eSlideManager and web gallery server storage repositories. This process produces a Deep Zoom image format file to organize a related set of directories containing pyramid image tiles as JPEG image files.

The dealer protocol, used to distribute batches of SVS image conversion tasks by eSlideManager database ImageID value, is an innovation developed within the MBRC to generate multiple Deep Zoom images in parallel, with the parallelization occurring within and across a fleet of virtual servers. The architecture is scalable by design. Additional storage and working memory capacity would enable more concurrent image conversion tasks per server. Additional servers in the image conversion server fleet would further expand concurrent image conversion capacity. When image conversion is complete, Deep Zoom images are copied from the virtual image conversion server to the web gallery server storage repository to enable public access. Files related to the image conversion process are removed from the image conversion servers after a successful copy to long-term storage is completed between rounds of image conversion. The system components and relationships of the MBRC image conversion pipeline from Aperio SVS images to Deep Zoom images are shown in **Figure 3**.

2.7.3 Digital output

MBRC web-accessible galleries generally display dozens of Deep Zoom images in a custom-built, responsive, labeled image frame template. The International Image Interoperability Framework (IIIF) is a set of open standards for delivering high-quality, attributed digital objects online at scale [18]. Deep Zoom images can

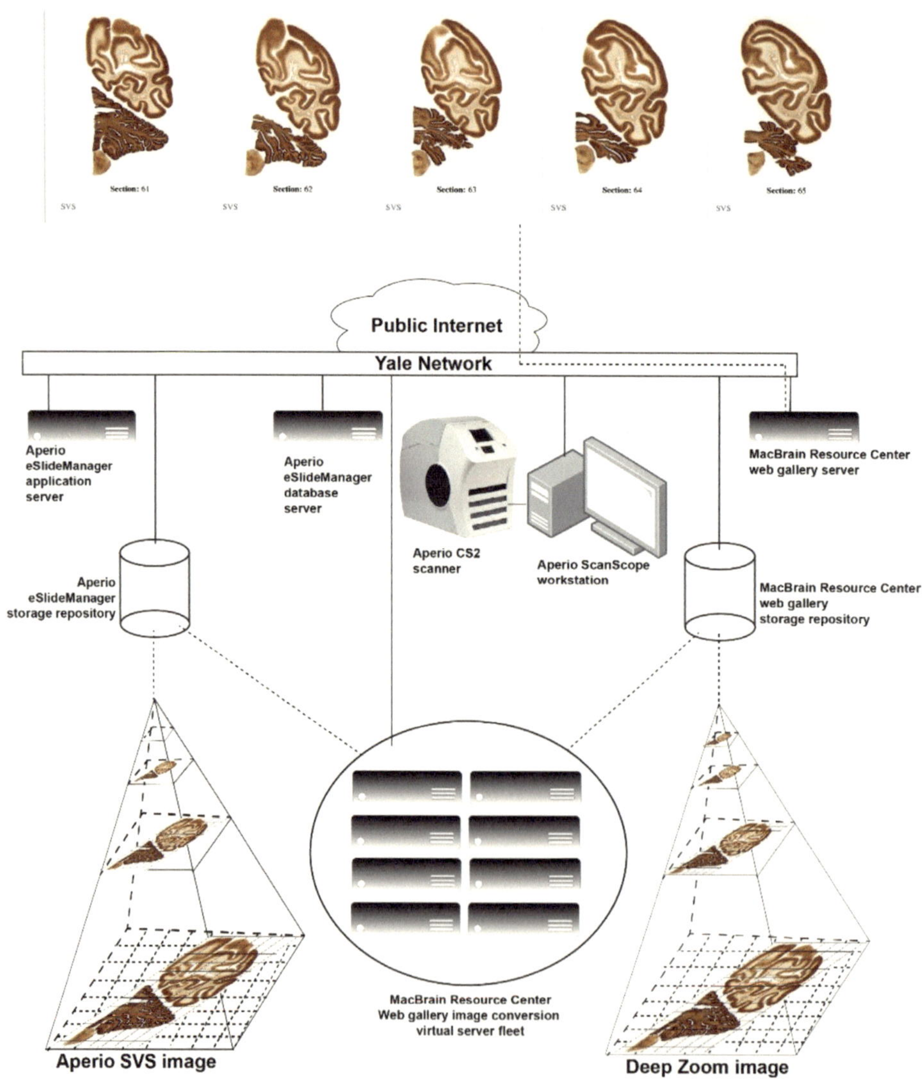

Figure 3.
MacBrain Resource Center (MBRC) image conversion pipeline from Aperio SVS images to Deep Zoom images.

be displayed with IIIF viewers. Seadragon software, the original developer of the Deep Zoom image format, formerly Sand Codex software, was acquired by Microsoft in 2006. OpenSeaDragon is an IIIF image viewer capable of displaying Deep Zoom images [19]. Based on Microsoft's open-source Seadragon Ajax library, MBRC web galleries include JavaScript-based OpenSeaDragon viewer components arranged in a responsive grid to display Deep Zoom, a set of images in each of our web galleries, enabling public access from a range of devices to, at the time of writing, over 30,000 full-resolution, zoomable whole-slide images of over 30 different neuronal and glia markers of 30 NHP brains of diverse age and sex. All images are accessible without plugins or logins, zoomable, and downloadable (**Figure 4**).

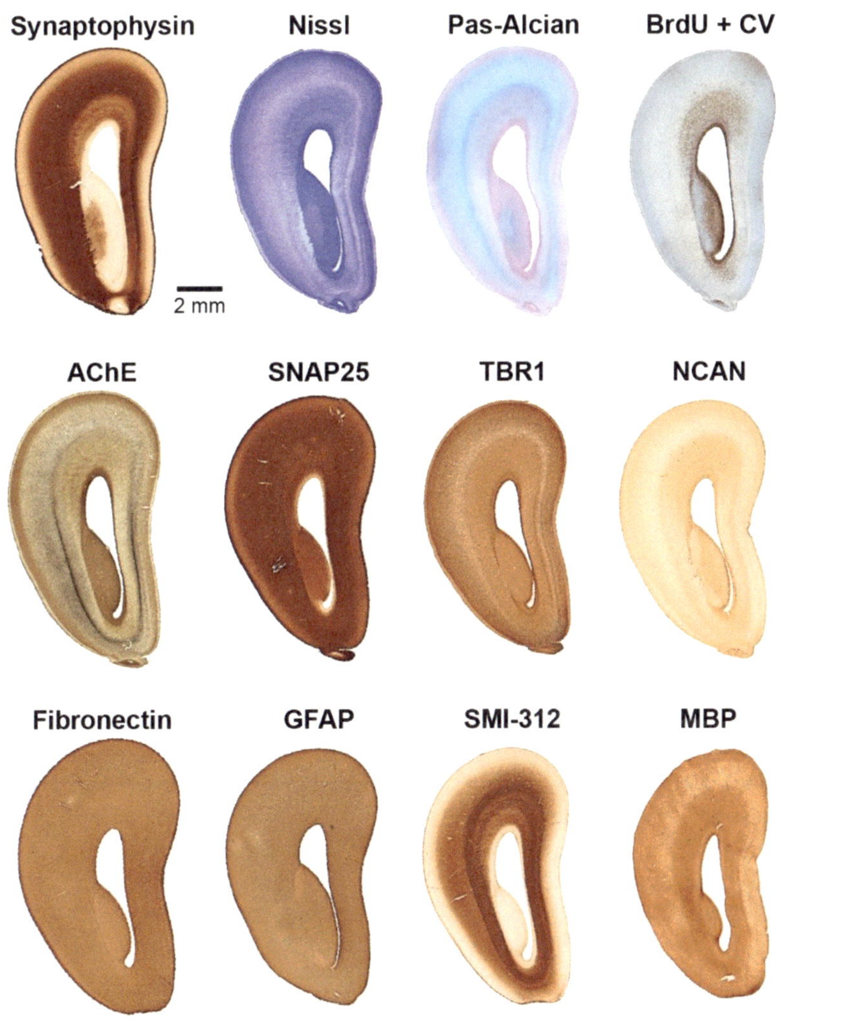

Figure 4.
Histo- and immunohistochemistry of a series of sections stained with different markers. Raw data to study developmental changes. Here, 12 different markers at embryonic age 70 (E70). Gestation in rhesus macaques is on average 165 days. Abbreviations: Periodic Acid-Schiff (PAS)-Alcian blue stain (Pas-Alcian), Bromodeoxyuridine counterstained with cresyl violet (BrdU+CV), acetylcholinesterase (AChE), 25 kDa Synaptosomal-Associated Protein (SNAP25), brain specific T-box transcription factor 1 (TBR1), Neurocan (NCAN), Glial fibrillary acidic protein (GFAP), Pan-axonal Phosphorylated neurofilament protein (SMI-312), and myelin basic protein (MBP). The scale bar applies to all images. Coronal sections of the left hemisphere were cut at 30-micron thickness.

2.8 Leveraging machine learning for NHP brain developmental studies

The rapid expansion of biomedical data, driven by advancements in neuroimaging, electrophysiology, and omics technologies, presents unprecedented opportunities to enhance patient care, deepen disease understanding, and refine treatment strategies [20, 21]. However, conventional analytical approaches, constrained by predefined rules and manual feature selection, frequently struggle to discern the complex patterns embedded within the extensive biomedical datasets [22, 23]. Machine learning (ML) is revolutionizing neuroscience by automating complex data analysis, enabling pattern recognition, and enhancing predictive modeling, thereby increasing research accuracy and efficiency [23–27]. The MBRC, as a primary repository of nonhuman primate (NHP) brain data, presents substantial opportunities for ML investigations into brain development, structural organization, and disease pathology [28]. Integrating ML techniques with MBRC's datasets could yield novel insights into primate brain function and advance neuroscience research.

Despite the wealth of available brain data, conventional statistical methods often fall short of capturing the intricate and nonlinear characteristics inherent in these datasets [29]. Traditional approaches, predicated on predefined assumptions, feature selection, and representative samples, may prove inadequate for extensive datasets. While classical techniques like principal component analysis (PCA) or support vector machines (SVMs) handle specific aspects of high-dimensional data, their scalability for nonlinear interactions remains limited without ML enhancements [30–32]. By contrast, ML uncovers hidden relationships and excels in capturing complex, implicit associations [33]. This capability is particularly evident in deep-learning architectures like convolutional neural networks (CNNs), which have successfully extracted meaningful patterns from immunohistochemistry (IHC) images. For instance, researchers developed LaceDNN, a deep-learning model that improves protein subcellular localization by leveraging label correlations [34]. Similarly, CNNs have shown promise in clinical diagnostics, significantly enhancing the identification of u-serrated patterns in direct immunofluorescence (DIF) microscopy images, a key marker for diagnosing epidermolysis bullosa acquisita [35]. Furthermore, researchers have used CNNs to automatically annotate gene expression patterns in developing mouse brains, outperforming traditional text-derived methods and showcasing the potential of transfer learning in large-scale biological image analysis [36].

The MBRC is pioneering low-cost methods to facilitate brain research by leveraging existing materials. As its collections continue to grow, ML presents a promising opportunity to enhance their utility [37]. ML can streamline key histological analyses within the MBRC, automating tasks such as cell segmentation, protein expression quantification, and tissue classification [38–41]. By reducing human error and significantly accelerating data processing, ML enables more efficient and scalable analysis of vast, high-dimensional datasets [33]. Unlike predefined statistical models, ML discerns complex patterns from data, mapping inputs to outcomes in ways that frequently generalize effectively to unseen cases, contingent on factors such as training data quality, regularization techniques, and model interpretability [29]. This capability renders ML especially valuable for revealing intricate relationships in histopathological data derived from NHP tissue samples. This ability to reveal previously unrecognized cellular and molecular patterns enhances the scientific value of MBRC's broad data archives. By prioritizing prediction and discovery, ML strengthens medical research, amplifying the impact of MBRC's collections in neuroscience.

2.9 Examples of data analysis, combining old and new materials and techniques

Many of the archived materials in the MBRC collections were procured and processed decades ago (e.g., materials in Collections 1 and 5), and a lot of newly processed materials are constantly added (e.g., the expanding Collections 6 and 7). Together, the materials complement each other, therefore avoiding unnecessary repetition of procedures already carried out and unnecessary animal sacrifice. Plenty of *de novo* research has already been published re-mining old materials using newer techniques [6, 7, 9, 42–44]. Below are a few examples of ongoing research taking advantage of these very unique strengths.

2.9.1 Example of de novo research into the genesis of choroid plexus using tritiated thymidine

Despite the importance of the choroid plexus in the production of cerebrospinal fluid (CSF) and the diagnostic importance of CSF itself, information on the kinetics of choroid plexus genesis is extremely scarce. We are currently investigating choroid plexus generation and development by following its evolution in the lateral and 4th ventricles of the developing NHP brain using samples from NHPs exposed to tritiated thymidine (^{3}H-TdR) at different embryonic ages and that were sacrificed at different intervals after injection, including postnatally. Positive cells are being detected by a host of methodologies. The ^{3}H-TdR was developed and visualized by autoradiography in the 1970s. The materials are available in Collection 1 of the MBRC (**Figure 5**).

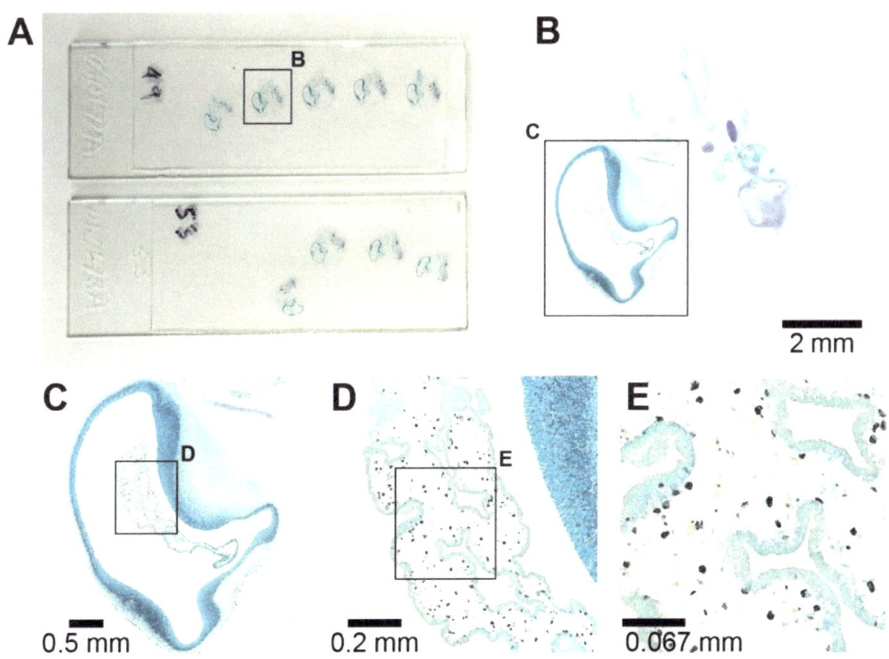

Figure 5.
Two glass slides containing nine coronal sections of embryonic macaque brain tissue (A). The pregnant NHP was injected with ^{3}H-TdR at E41, and the embryo was obtained by C-section and sacrificed an hour later. Sections were processed by autoradiography to reveal labeling of dividing cells at the time of injection and counterstained with Nissl to facilitate observation of landmarks (A–E). This specimen, in MBRC Collection 1, was obtained and processed on June 6, 1973 (hence case number 060673A). Sequentially zoomed-in views of the choroid plexus and surrounding lateral ventricle, highlighting the appearance and strength of silver labeling (B–E).

2.9.2 Example of de novo electron microscopy research of the developing neocortex

Collection 5 of the MBRC consists of thousands of brain tissue segments from NHP embryos of different ages, embedded in epoxy resin and suitable for electron microscopy analysis. **Figure 6** exemplifies materials being analyzed to continue studies of the kinetics of mammalian cerebral cortex expansion. Here, a 55-day-old monkey embryo brain was fixed and embedded in epoxy resin in May 1985. After 40 years of storage, the ultrastructure is perfectly sharp, and the specimen is appropriate for ultrathin sectioning and electron microscopy study, including 3-D reconstruction from serial sections. Some aspects of the long-term research on NHP brain development using Collection 5 of the MBRC have already been published [44–46].

2.9.3 Example of ML at work for the detection of striatal cholinergic interneurons

Figures 7 and **8** illustrate an in-house project that uses histological scans of an E110 female rhesus macaque brain embryo analyzed with an AI-driven tool, a commercially available image analysis software called Aiforia® Create, which enables researchers

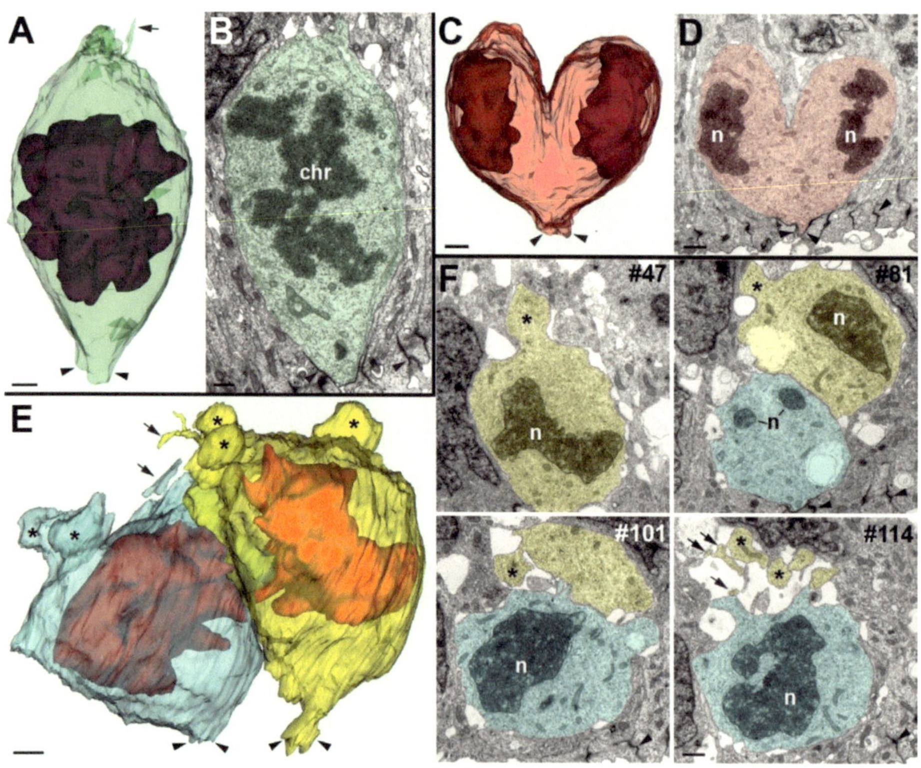

Figure 6.
Electron microscopy 3-D reconstruction from serial ultrathin sections of three mitotic cells in the neocortical ventricular zone of a 55-day-old rhesus macaque embryo. The emergence of condensed chromosomes in the cytoplasm or two opposing daughter nuclei shows that one cell is in metaphase (A, B), the other is in early cytokinesis (C, D), and the third is in late cytokinesis (E, F). Notice that these cells do not have radial processes but thin filopodia (arrows) or short protrusions of the cell membrane (asterisks). The reconstructed cells and their characteristic micrographs are highlighted with corresponding semitransparent colors (green, red, blue, and yellow). Chromosomes (chr) and daughter nuclei (n) are shown inside the cell bodies. The order of the micrographs in the series is indicated by the numbers in (F). The ventricular surface is identifiable with the row of adherens junctions that are indicated with arrowheads. Scale bars are 1 micron.

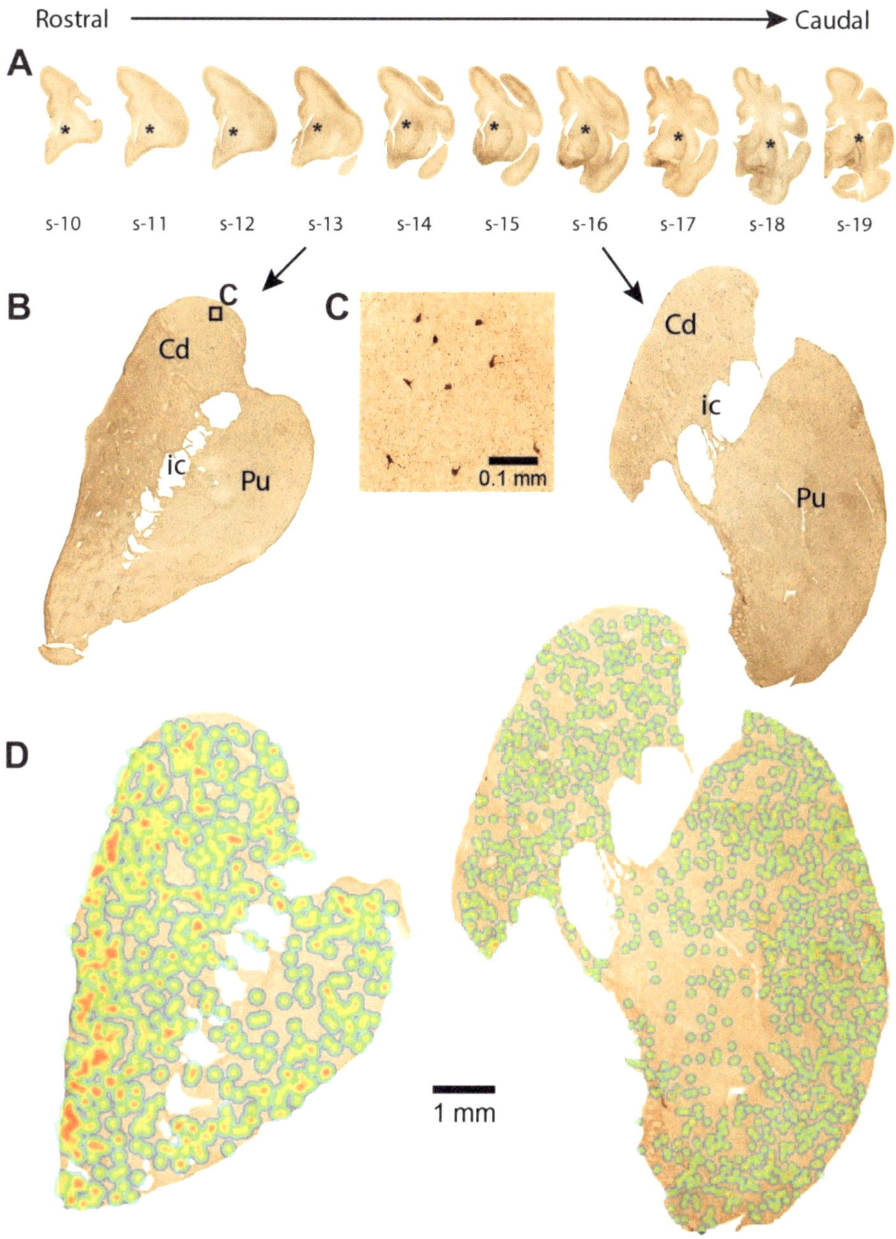

Figure 7.
Process for analyzing striatum in a female rhesus macaque embryo, age: E110. Images of all sections containing striatum are collected for analysis, one hemisphere, rostral-to-caudal (A). The image of each section is edited to contain only the striatum: Caudate and putamen (B). ChAT+ cells within the striatal area are clearly distinguishable at higher magnification (C). After training, Aiforia detects cells, producing a density heatmap (D) and downloadable quantitative data.

to develop ML models tailored to their own research questions. The interface does not require familiarity with written code, only annotations on a set of training images. This technology demonstrates a methodology to mine (and re-mine) existing digital material for new insights into the cytoarchitecture of the NHP brain. Although this example is from a study focused on cholinergic interneurons in the striatum of female

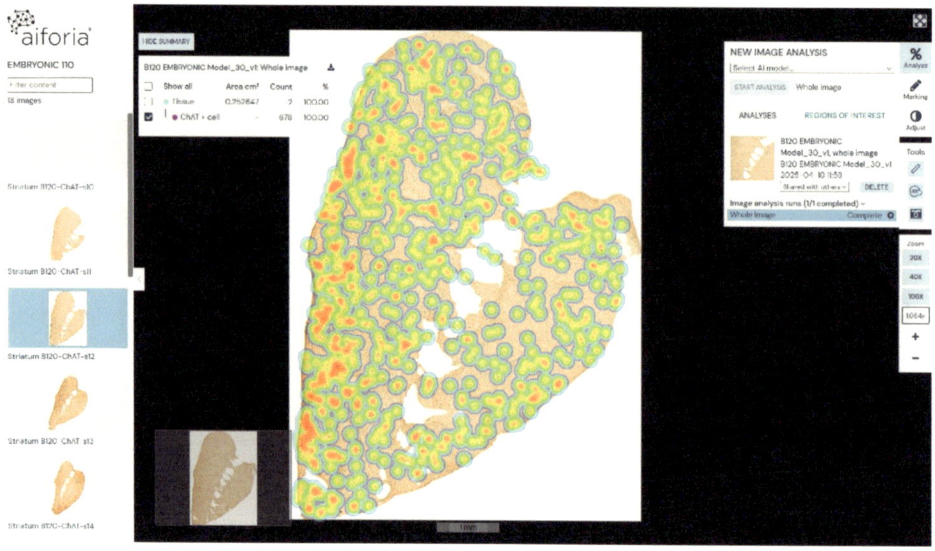

Figure 8.
View of the Aiforia interface after performing image analysis. Results are visualized in a zoomable heat map; quantifications of tissue area and cell counts are summarized on screen, with the option to download a detailed Excel spreadsheet. E110. Serial interactions of ML-based training ensure the algorithm is then able to detect and measure cells very quickly and with a very high level of confidence.

NHPs, the same method can and will be used to detect, count, and measure other features in other regions of the brain and in males. This is an example of tissue from Collection 7 that was specifically processed for ChAT immunohistochemistry, which is then detected and analyzed using ML/AI technology. The materials under study will then be incorporated into Collection 6 and become publicly available.

3. Conclusions

The goal of this chapter has been to raise awareness of the need for and importance of establishing reliable datasets for the study of NHP brain development and to introduce the collections available in the MBRC that can contribute to these efforts. As useful as MRI and other imaging techniques have been, and will continue to be, histology is unsurpassed in studies of cytoarchitecture because of its cellular resolution. We advocate the need to increase the sharing of resources to increase the number of available samples for study. Proper and complete documentation of the samples and of the processing parameters is absolutely necessary to assure usefulness without compromising scientific rigor. We consider the establishment of reliable NHP brain development datasets essential to advance the fields of neurodevelopment and neuroscience, and we have started to process tissue to populate the already established Collection 6 of the MBRC with such materials.

Acknowledgements

This work is supported by NIH grant MH113257 (AD). Studies that contributed embryonic brain hemispheres and blocks to the MBRC are supported largely by DA023999 (PR).

Conflict of interest

The authors declare no conflict of interest.

Notes/thanks/other declarations

We thank Ashley Ake, Esmeralda Alejo, Mari Elliott, and Mikhail Rodov for scanning materials for analysis.

Author details

Alvaro Duque*, Phil Barello, Lucy Greene, Emma Burke, Valeria Mendoza-Silva, Yury M. Morozov and Pasko Rakic
Department of Neuroscience, MacBrain Resource Center, Yale University School of Medicine, New Haven, CT, USA

*Address all correspondence to: alvaro.duque@yale.edu

References

[1] Mitsunaga F, Ueiwa M, Kamanaka Y, Morimoto M, Nakamura S. Fetal sex determination of macaque monkeys by a nested PCR using maternal plasma. Experimental Animals. 2010;**59**(2):255-260

[2] Junaković A, Kopić J, Duque A, Rakic P, Krsnik Ž, Kostović I. Laminar dynamics of deep projection neurons and mode of subplate formation are hallmarks of histogenetic subdivisions of the human cingulate cortex before onset of arealization. Brain Structure & Function. 20230102nd ed. 2023;**228**(2):613-633

[3] Li H, Duque A, Rakic P. Origin and development of the claustrum in rhesus macaque. Proceedings of the National Academy of Sciences of the United States of America. 20230705th ed. 2023;**120**(28):e2220918120

[4] Micali N, Ma S, Li M, Kim SK, Mato-Blanco X, Sindhu SK, et al. Molecular programs of regional specification and neural stem cell fate progression in macaque telencephalon. Science. 20231013th ed. 2023;**382**(6667):eadf3786

[5] Rash BG, Arellano JI, Duque A, Rakic P. Role of intracortical neuropil growth in the gyrification of the primate cerebral cortex. Proceedings of the National Academy of Sciences of the United States of America. 20221227th ed. 2023;**120**(1):e2210967120

[6] Sakharkar M, Rockland KS, Duque A. Complex neurochemical microstructure of the stria terminalis in infant and adult macaque monkey. Frontiers in Neuroanatomy. 20220525th ed. 2022;**16**:891608

[7] McDonald AJ, Duque A. Specific neuronal subpopulations in the amygdala of macaque monkeys express high levels of nonphosphorylated neurofilaments. Brain Research. 20211224th ed. 2022;**1777**:147767

[8] Rash BG, Duque A, Morozov YM, Arellano JI, Micali N, Rakic P. Gliogenesis in the outer subventricular zone promotes enlargement and gyrification of the primate cerebrum. Proceedings of the National Academy of Sciences of the United States of America. 20190320th ed. 2019;**116**(14):7089-7094

[9] Duque A, Krsnik Z, Kostović I, Rakic P. Secondary expansion of the transient subplate zone in the developing cerebrum of human and nonhuman primates. Proceedings of the National Academy of Sciences of the United States of America. 20160808th ed. 2016;**113**(35):9892-9897

[10] Duque A, Gazula VR, Kaczmarek LK. Expression of Kv1.3 potassium channels regulates density of cortical interneurons. Developmental Neurobiology. 20130911th ed. 2013;**73**(11):841-855

[11] Duque A, Tepper JM, Detari L, Ascoli GA, Zaborszky L. Morphological characterization of electrophysiologically and immunohistochemically identified basal forebrain cholinergic and neuropeptide Y-containing neurons. Brain Structure & Function. 20070602nd ed. 2007;**212**(1):55-73

[12] Duque A, Balatoni B, Detari L, Zaborszky L. EEG correlation of the discharge properties of identified neurons in the basal forebrain. Journal of Neurophysiology. 2000;**84**(3):1627-1635

[13] Hsu SM, Raine L, Fanger H. Use of avidin-biotin-peroxidase complex (ABC)

in immunoperoxidase techniques: A comparison between ABC and unlabeled antibody (PAP) procedures. The Journal of Histochemistry and Cytochemistry. 1981;**29**(4):577-580

[14] Hsu SM, Raine L. Protein A, avidin, and biotin in immunohistochemistry. The Journal of Histochemistry and Cytochemistry. 1981;**29**(11):1349-1353

[15] Aperio Technologies Inc. Digital Slides and Third-Party Data Interchange [Internet]. Vista, CA, United States; 2008. Available from: http://www.aperio.com/documents/api/Aperio_Digital_Slides_and_Third-party_data_interchange.pdf [Accessed: March 6, 2025]

[16] Balkan A. OpenSlide [Internet]. 2013. Available from: https://openslide.org/ [Accessed: March 6, 2025]

[17] Microsoft. Deep Zoom File Format Overview [Internet]. 2011. Available from: https://learn.microsoft.com/en-us/previous-versions/windows/silverlight/dotnet-windows-silverlight/cc645077(v=vs.95)?redirectedfrom=MSDN [Accessed: March 6, 2025]

[18] Framework III. How it Works [Internet]. Available from: https://iiif.io/get-started/how-iiif-works/ [Accessed: March 6, 2025]

[19] Project O. DZI Tile Source [Internet]. Available from: https://openseadragon.github.io/examples/tilesource-dzi/ [Accessed: March 6, 2025]

[20] Ngiam KY, Khor IW. Big data and machine learning algorithms for health-care delivery. The Lancet Oncology. 2019;**20**(5):e262-e273

[21] Prosperi M, Min JS, Bian J, Modave F. Big data hurdles in precision medicine and precision public health. BMC Medical Informatics and Decision Making. 2018;**18**(1):139

[22] Huang X, Li Z, Zhang M, Gao S. Fusing hand-crafted and deep-learning features in a convolutional neural network model to identify prostate cancer in pathology images. Frontiers in Oncology. 20220927th ed. 2022;**12**:994950

[23] Zhang J, Xia Y, Xie Y, Fulham MJ, Feng DD. Classification of medical images in the biomedical literature by jointly using deep and handcrafted visual features. IEEE Journal of Biomedical and Health Informatics. 2018;**22**:1521-1530

[24] Cascarano A, Mur-Petit J, Hernández-González J, Camacho M, Eadie N, Gkontra P, et al. Machine and deep learning for longitudinal biomedical data: A review of methods and applications. Artificial Intelligence Review. 2023;**56**:1711-1771

[25] Seo H, Badiei Khuzani M, Vasudevan V, Huang C, Ren H, Xiao R, et al. Machine learning techniques for biomedical image segmentation: An overview of technical aspects and introduction to state-of-art applications. Medical Physics. 2020;**47**(5):e148-e167

[26] Delli Priscoli M, Memmolo P, Ciaparrone G, Bianco V, Merola F, Miccio L, et al. Neuroblastoma cells classification through learning approaches by direct analysis of digital holograms. IEEE Journal of Selected Topics in Quantum Electronics. 2021;**27**:1-9

[27] Buchlak QD, Esmaili N, Leveque JCA, Farrokhi FR, Bennett CC, Piccardi M, et al. Machine learning applications to clinical decision support in neurosurgery: An artificial intelligence augmented systematic review. Neurosurgical Review. 2019;**43**:1235-1253

[28] Duque A. Reducing Non-Human Primate Sacrifice for Brain Research in the Virtual Era [Internet]. Open Access Government; 2023. Available from: https://www.openaccessgovernment.org/reducing-non-human-primate-sacrifice-for-brain-research-in-the-virtual-era/170646/

[29] Rajula HSR, Verlato G, Manchia M, Antonucci N, Fanos V. Comparison of conventional statistical methods with machine learning in medicine: Diagnosis, drug development, and treatment. Medicina (Kaunas). 20200908th ed. 8 Sep 2020;**56**(9):1-10

[30] Morishita T. Time-dependent principal component analysis: A unified approach to high-dimensional data reduction using adiabatic dynamics. The Journal of Chemical Physics. 2021;**155**(13):134114

[31] Kramer MA. Nonlinear principal component analysis using autoassociative neural networks. AICHE Journal. 1991;**37**:233-243

[32] Li B, Artemiou A, Li L. Principal support vector machines for linear and nonlinear sufficient dimension reduction. Annals of Statistics. 2011;**39**:3182-3210

[33] Sidey-Gibbons JAM, Sidey-Gibbons CJ. Machine learning in medicine: A practical introduction. BMC Medical Research Methodology. 20190319th ed. 2019;**19**(1):64

[34] Hu JX, Yang Y, Xu YY, Shen H. Incorporating label correlations into deep neural networks to classify protein subcellular location patterns in immunohistochemistry images. Proteins: Structure. 2021;**90**:493-503

[35] Shi C, Meijer JM, Azzopardi G, Diercks GFH, Guo J, Petkov N. Use of convolutional neural networks for the detection of u-serrated patterns in direct immunofluorescence images to facilitate the diagnosis of epidermolysis bullosa acquisita. The American Journal of Pathology. 20210628th ed. 2021;**191**(9):1520-1525

[36] Zeng T, Li R, Mukkamala R, Ye J, Ji S. Deep convolutional neural networks for annotating gene expression patterns in the mouse brain. BMC Bioinformatics. 2015;**16**(1):147

[37] Duque A. Fostering nonhuman primate (NHP) brain research without animal sacrifice. Open Access Government. 2023;**38**:186-186. DOI: 10.56367/OAG-038-10792

[38] Kan A. Machine learning applications in cell image analysis. Immunology and Cell Biology. 20170315th ed. 2017;**95**(6):525-530

[39] Durkee MS, Abraham R, Clark MR, Giger ML. Artificial intelligence and cellular segmentation in tissue microscopy images. The American Journal of Pathology. 2021;**191**(10):1693-1701

[40] Claeys T, Menu M, Bouwmeester R, Gevaert K, Martens L. Machine learning on large-scale proteomics data identifies tissue and cell-type specific proteins. Journal of Proteome Research. 2022;**22**:1181-1192

[41] Rączkowski Ł, Możejko M, Zambonelli J, Szczurek E. ARA: Accurate, reliable and active histopathological image classification framework with Bayesian deep learning. Scientific Reports. 2019;**9**(1):1-12

[42] Spadory T, Duque A, Selemon L. Spatial-temporal topography in neurogenesis of the macaque thalamus.

Brain Structure and Function. 2022;**227**(5):1673-1682

[43] Ahmed B, Duque A, Rakic P, Molnár Z. Correlation between the number of interstitial neurons of the white matter and number of neurons within cortical layers: Histological analyses in postnatal macaque. The Journal of Comparative Neurology. 2024;**532**(6):e25626

[44] Morozov YM, Rakic P. Lateral expansion of the mammalian cerebral cortex is related to anchorage of centrosomes in apical neural progenitors. Cerebral Cortex. 3 Jul 2024;**34**(7):1-9

[45] Morozov YM, Mackie K, Rakic P. Cannabinoid type 1 receptor is undetectable in rodent and primate cerebral neural stem cells but participates in radial neuronal migration. International Journal of Molecular Sciences. 20201117th ed. 17 Nov 2020;**21**(22):1-19

[46] Arellano JI, Morozov YM, Micali N, Rakic P. Radial glial cells: New views on old questions. Neurochemical Research. 20210316th ed. 2021;**46**(10):2512-2524

Chapter 6

The Impact of Hemichannel-Mediated Neuroinflammation at Early Stages of CNS Ontogeny in the Development of Adult Neuropsychiatric Diseases

Francisco J. Ocaranza and Juan C. Sáez

Abstract

In pathological conditions, elevated activity of connexin and pannexin hemichannels facilitates adenosine triphosphate (ATP) efflux and Ca^{2+} influx, activating metabolic pathways of neuroinflammation. While a small insult could result in a protective inflammatory response, more intense and/or prolonged insults induce cell death, causing tissue dysfunction. In the brain, different stressors elevate glucocorticoid (GC) levels that are sensed by mast cells and microglia, and this response persists for a long time, causing continuous inflammasome activation and release of IL-1β and IL-18. These proinflammatory cytokines, together with those released by mast cells, activate astrocytes and oligodendrocytes, which in turn release glutamate and ATP, and altogether reduce neuronal functionality and survival. The extent of neuroinflammation also depends on host features that result in different degrees of alterations during brain ontogeny, consequently changing the brain cytoarchitecture and leading to spectrums of behavioral diseases. Selective hemichannel blockers have been recently discovered and shown to reduce neuroinflammation, as well as neuronal suffering and symptoms linked to adult models of depression and epilepsy. These blockers can serve as tools to dissect the role of neuroinflammation in behavioral diseases. Early treatment during brain ontogeny could reduce detrimental impacts on the brain cytoarchitecture, inducing behavioral alterations elicited in adulthood.

Keywords: stress, gestation, connexons, pannexons, glial cell activation, proliferation, differentiation, anti-inflammatory, large-pore channels

1. Introduction

In the nervous system, inflammation is called neuroinflammation and can be local, incipient, massive, or chronic, being highly dependent on two main factors:

insult and subject characteristics. Insults can be categorized by intensity (quantity or amount), duration (time and frequency), and quality (location and condition where the stimulus is received). There can also be combinations of different insult features that could induce different neuroinflammatory responses in the same individual. Furthermore, the intrinsic characteristics of the individual receiving the insult also influence the outcomes of the neuroinflammatory response. These intrinsic characteristics include age, sex, hormonal and feeding status, preexisting and pharmacological conditions, and phenotypic changes induced by circadian and seasonal rhythms. In addition, during gestation, the mother's health conditions (e.g., preeclampsia, diabetes) [1] and environmental insults (e.g., viral, bacterial, or parasitic infections; smoke; alcohol; drug abuse; radiation; toxic compounds; psychological and physical abuse) can cause neuroinflammation in the offspring. Notably, neuroinflammation that unfolds during brain ontogeny is directly associated with neuropsychiatric conditions in adults, according to human and animal models [2–4]. However, direct

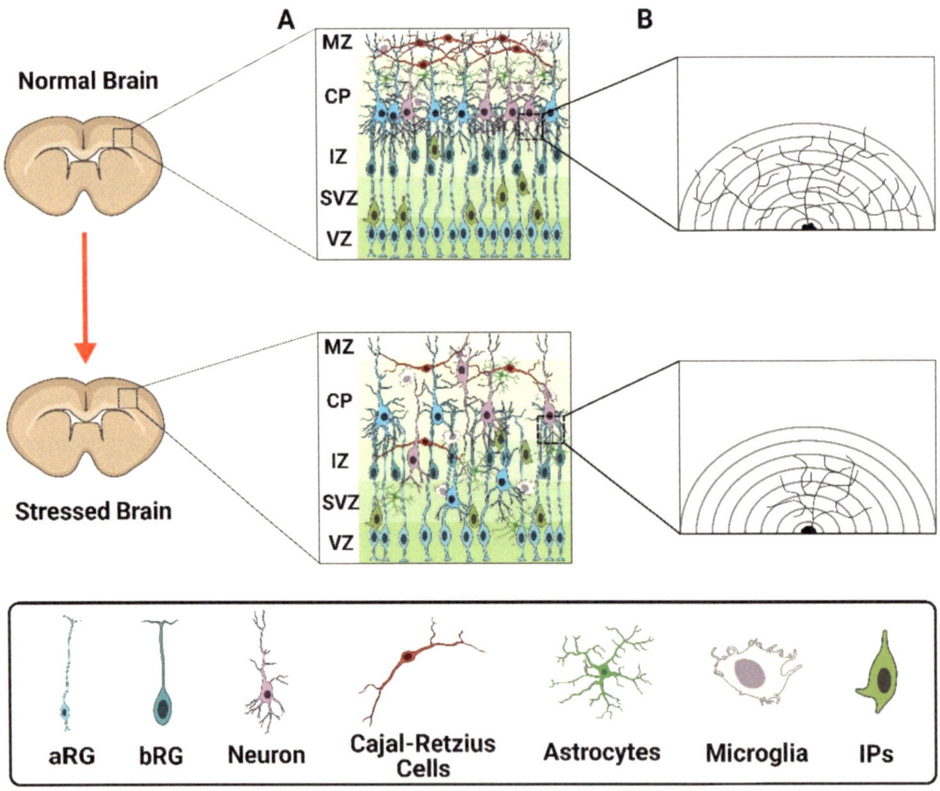

Figure 1.
Scheme of cellular distribution in the embryonic neocortex during central nervous system (CNS) development and dendritic arborization of a neuron between a normal and a stressed brain **(A)** *Scheme of the distribution of glia and neurons during brain development in mice; above, illustration of a normal brain and the proper distribution of the different cell types in the ventricular zone (VZ), subventricular zone (SVZ), intermediate zone (IZ), cortical plate (CP), and marginal zone (MZ); below, illustration of the same zones and distribution of the cells in a stressed brain, showing changes in the placement of all types of cells and changes in arborization of neurons [7].* **(B)** *Scheme of dendritic arborization marked with Golgi-Cox staining. The neuron of a stressed brain (below) shows fewer neuronal intersections and shorter dendrite lengths compared to the neuron of a normal brain (above) [8]. Images obtained and adapted from NIH BIOART, Source [9–11], and/or created by the authors based on the published bibliography. All images were created, modified, and assembled on Inkscape (https://inkscape.org/).*

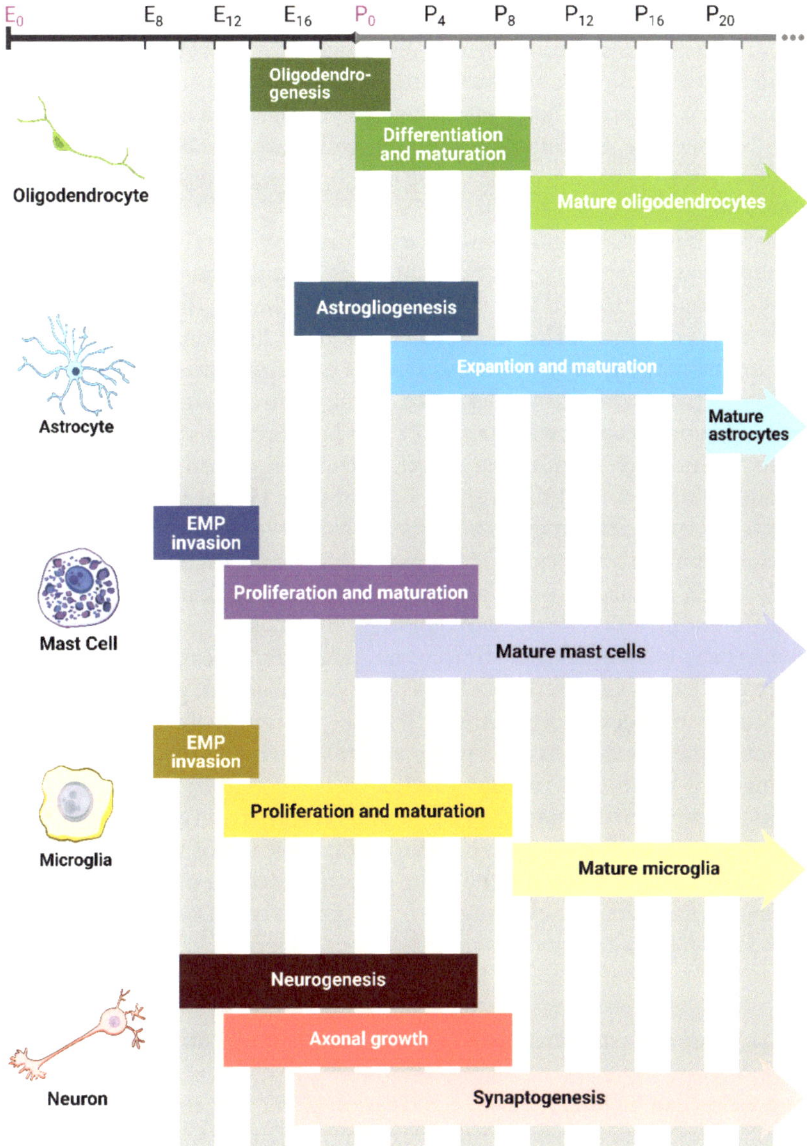

Figure 2.
Timeline of the ontogeny of CNS cells. In order to start from the top, oligodendrocytes start to appear on embryonic day (E) 14; the genesis of the oligodendrocytes lasts until postnatal day (P) 2, and just before this day, P0 initiates the maturation and differentiation of the oligodendrocytes, resulting in mature oligodendrocytes, which emerge around P9 [12–14]. Astrocyte genesis starts around E16.5, ending on P7. On day P2, the new astrocytes start to expand and mature, ending around day P21, when the mature astrocytes appear in the CNS [12, 14–16]. Mast cells and microglia originate from the bone marrow and enter the brain during development, starting with the invasion of the erythroid-myeloid progenitor (EMP) from the yolk sac through the circulatory system that is being generated at the same time. This invasion starts around day E8.5 and ends on day E14 to E15. On day E12.5, the maturation and proliferation of both cell types occur with little difference in the time of ending and the appearance of the mature cell types. In mast cells, the proliferation and maturation phases end around day P7, while microglia extend these processes to about day P9. Mature mast cells appear around day P0, while mature microglia take a little longer, emerging around day P9 [12, 17, 18]. Finally, neurons in the hippocampus start their ontogeny on day E10, ending on day P7, while axonal growth of new neurons starts almost in conjunction with their genesis, initiating on day E12.5 and ending on day P9. Synaptogenesis starts on day E16.5 and is a continuous process in the CNS [12, 16, 19]. Images were obtained and adapted from SciDraw [20–24] and/or created by the authors based on the published bibliography. All images were created, adapted, and assembled on Inkscape (https://inkscape.org/).

cause-and-effect evidence of the role of neuroinflammation in causing tissue dysfunctions remains elusive, and thus far, therapies for even the most chronic brain diseases do not include treatment with anti-neuroinflammatory agents. The ultimate action of inflammation is to restore homeostasis in affected tissues with high regeneration capacity [5]. Otherwise, the outcome would be cell death that could lead to tissue dysfunction when the number of surviving cells is not sufficient to perform proficient tissue functions.

To understand the etiopathogenesis of numerous psychiatric conditions, such as neurodevelopmental disorders, it is relevant to identify the developmental stage at which an individual is affected by a specific insult. In theory, the same insult received at different stages of intrauterine life or early postnatal life would have distinct outcomes in the ontogeny of the nervous system. Emerging studies also reveal that the gut microbiome plays a relevant role in modulating neuroinflammatory conditions [6]. These differences could be explained in part by alterations at critical steps of brain development, such as induction, proliferation, migration, or differentiation of glia and neurons that occur at different periods of time (**Figures 1** and **2**). As a result, the normal developmental program is not achieved correctly. This could explain the multiple functional and structural alterations associated with behavioral changes [25, 26]. However, a cause-effect relationship remains to be demonstrated. A common factor of different insults is stress, which under physiological conditions is an adaptive response to an environmental stimulus perceived as "threatening." This stimulus, called a stressor, can have different origins (e.g., psychosocial, physical, chemical, or biological) and can affect an organism individually or jointly. A common response, independent of the stressor, involves glucocorticoids, which promote glial cell activation, causing long-lasting neuroinflammation [27].

In addition, neuroinflammation can be transferred to future generations through epigenetic mechanisms (see Section 6). The therapeutic use of new agents that revert molecular epigenetic signatures in the same generation could prevent their transfer to the following generation. The efficacy of this approach could be complemented with new anti-inflammatory compounds that block nonselective channels (see below).

2. Molecular aspects of neuroinflammation and anti-inflammatory agents

Inflammation can be induced by the activation of canonical and/or noncanonical pathways. The canonical pathway responds to stimuli from various immune receptors and leads to rapid but transient activation of NF-κB through the activation of TGFβ-activated kinase 1 (TAK1 or MAP3K7), which activates the trimeric IκB kinase complex (IKK). After several steps, the process culminates with the nuclear translocation of elements such as NF-κB1 p50, RELA, and c-REL, at which they bind to DNA at κB enhancer sites where they exert their action [28].

The noncanonical pathway is based on the processing of p100, which is tightly controlled and inducible. P100, also known as NF-κB2, is a precursor protein that, after processing, becomes the p52 subunit of the NF-κB transcription factor. Processing of p100 induces the translocation of p100-associated NF-κB family members such as RELB and NF-κB p52. One of the characteristics of this pathway is its slow and persistent activation, and its activation is mediated by ligands of tumor necrosis factor receptors (TNFRs), such as TNFα [28].

An overproduction of TNFα has been observed in rats subjected to acute stress by immobilization. TNFα is involved in the expression of inducible nitric oxide synthase

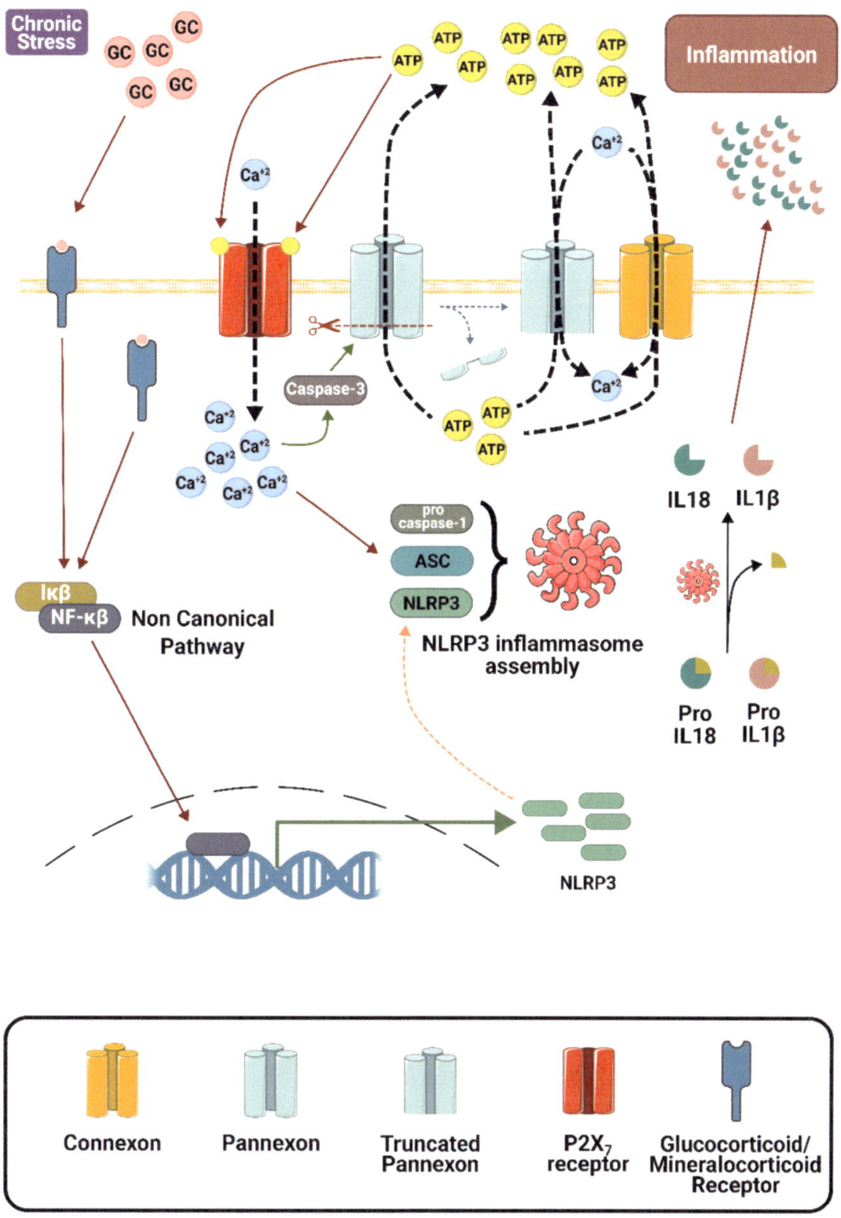

Figure 3.
Scheme of inflammasome activation and generation of an inflammatory environment in a cell. From left to right, a stress stimulus induces high levels of glucocorticoids (GCs), which bind to the mineralocorticoid or glucocorticoid receptors (MRs/GRs) in the cell membrane or cell lumen, activating the inflammatory pathway in a neighboring cell through the Iκβ/NF-κβ complex. This complex then induces the transcriptions and elevated levels of NLRP3. GCs also induce the release of ATP from mast cells, which binds to the P2X7 receptor, enabling the influx of Ca^{2+}. Elevated Ca^{2+} levels in the intracellular milieu enhance the activity of pannexin1 hemichannels (Pannexons), allowing for ATP to be released into the extracellular milieu, where the activity of connexin hemichannels (Connexons) enables the influx of Ca^{2+} and efflux of ATP. Similar ATP and Ca^{2+} transmembrane transfer occurs through truncated pannexons. Elevated levels of intracellular free Ca^{2+} also induce the assembly of NLRP3, ASC, and pro-caspase1, forming the NLRP3 inflammasome. This promotes cleavage of the proinflammatory cytokines pro-IL1β and pro-IL18 to their active forms. The subsequent release of these cytokines induces a local proinflammatory environment. Images above were obtained and adapted from NIH BIOART Source [34–36], Servier medical art [37–40], and/or created by the authors based on the published bibliography. All images were created, modified, and assembled in Inkscape (https://inkscape.org/).

(iNOS) through NF-κB-dependent mechanisms [29]. However, these changes are not the same in different brain areas. For instance, rats subjected to chronic stress show an increase in NF-κB activation as well as in the expression of TNFα, IL-1β, and iNOS in the hippocampus, but the opposite occurs in the hypothalamus [30].

Elevated levels of TNFα and ATP in the extracellular lumen have been linked to the assembly of the inflammasome, a 700 kDa protein complex responsible for the activation of the proinflammatory cytokines IL-1β and IL-18 [31, 32]. Our interest in this chapter is in the NLRP3 inflammasome, which is composed of the NOD-like receptor family pyrin domain containing 3 (NLRP3) protein as a sensor, the apoptosis-associated speck-like protein containing an activator and recruiter of the caspase domain as an adapter protein (ASC: apoptosis-associated speck-like protein containing a CARD), and the protease caspase-1 as an effector [31, 33].

The inflammasome can be activated by several stimuli and ligands, including pathogen-associated molecular patterns (PAMPs) and damage-associated molecular patterns (DAMPs), such as TNFα and ATP. The presence of TNFα in the extracellular lumen activates the TNF receptor (TNFR). This results in the upregulation of inactive NLRP3, which, together with the ASC protein, induces the autocatalysis of caspase-1 from pro-caspase-1, resulting in the cleavage of pro-IL-1β and pro-IL-18 to IL-1β and IL-18 (**Figure 3**) [31, 33, 41, 42]. Furthermore, IL-1β is known to act in a paracrine/autocrine manner, improving signaling in the hypothalamus-pituitary-adrenal axis during stress, which results in higher cytokine and glucocorticoid (GC) production [41].

The same effect on the activation of the inflammasome is achieved by ATP through the activation of the purinergic receptor P2X ligand-gated ion channel 7 (P2X7 receptor or P2X7R). Elevated levels of extracellular ATP activate the P2X7R, enabling the influx of Ca^{2+} into the intracellular milieu (**Figure 3**) [43, 44]. This elevation in cytoplasmic Ca^{2+} leads to two results. First, it activates connexin hemichannels (connexons) and cleavage of the C-terminal of pannexin1 by caspase-3. This generates a truncated pannexin1 hemichannel that, together with connexin and intact pannexin hemichannels, enhances ATP efflux to the extracellular milieu [45, 46], thus amplifying the inflammation signal. Second, Ca^{2+} elevation induces the upregulation of NLRP3, in an analogous manner to TNFα, also resulting in the activation of IL-1β and IL-18 (**Figure 3**) [31, 33, 42]. The NLRP3 inflammasome and its activation occur in most cell types of the central nervous system (CNS), including mast cells [42], microglia [47], astrocytes [48], oligodendrocytes [41, 49], and neurons [50].

If this inflammatory process occurs during the ontogeny of the nervous system, it can have significant undesired consequences, affecting processes such as microglial infiltration and expansion, neurogenesis, gliogenesis, connection generation, and neuronal pruning (**Figures 1** and **2**) [12]. Numerous anatomical studies have demonstrated that changes in neuronal structure and function are responsible for many of the stress-induced changes in behavior and cognition [51–53], opening a possible explanation for the etiopathogenesis of neuropsychiatric illnesses such as anxiety disorders and depression.

3. Stress and inflammation

The hypothalamus is involved in stress responses, activating a neuroendocrine response axis involving the pituitary and adrenal glands, called the hypothalamus-pituitary-adrenal axis. This axis receives information from the endocrine, immune, and nervous systems, controlling the physiological responses to stress [54].

The hypothalamus releases corticotropin-releasing hormone (CRH), which acts primarily on the pituitary gland, inducing the release of adrenocorticotropic hormone (ACTH), which ultimately induces the release of GCs from the adrenal cortex (cortisol in humans and corticosterone in rodents) [41, 54–56].

GCs coordinate the regulation of the circadian rhythm, with elevated levels during the first hours of the day and low points around midnight in humans [57–59]. This pattern is reversed in nocturnal organisms such as mice. Due to their lipophilic characteristics, GCs passively cross the plasma membrane of cells, where they can bind to the glucocorticoid receptor (GR) or the mineralocorticoid receptor (MR), with GR being a low-affinity receptor and MR a high-affinity receptor for GCs. The ligand-receptor complex is translocated to the nucleus, where it activates or represses the transcription of multiple genes [54, 60, 61]. This GC signaling pathway has been estimated to regulate up to 20% of the genome [54, 62], and therefore, they have multiple undesired effects on the brain and peripheral tissues.

The regulation of GC at the intracellular level depends on the activity of two 11β-hydroxysteroid dehydrogenase isoenzymes, which have opposite effects. While isoenzyme 2 (11β-HSD2) inactivates cortisol (or corticosterone) in (11β-HSDs), transforming it into cortisone (or 11-dehydrocorticosterone), isoenzyme 1 (11β-HSD1) activates GCs [63–65]. At the systemic level, GCs are regulated through corticosteroid-binding globulin, which in humans leaves approximately 5% cortisol circulating in its active form [64]. In addition to the canonical function of GCs, other mechanisms have been described where GCs exert their action, including non-genomic effects of GRs, as well as crosstalk with other transcription factors and GC effects that are receptor-independent [54, 66].

GC levels increase in response to stress, heightening the individual's state of alert and enabling a positive adaptive response to the stressor in cases of acute stress [67]. However, chronic stress happens to be proinflammatory in the CNS, where different cells of the immune system, such as mast cells and microglia, are activated, hence inducing a reactive state in astrocytes and oligodendrocytes. Just 30 minutes of movement restriction is enough for corticosterone to increase and mast cell degranulation to occur [68, 69], resulting in the release of proinflammatory agents such as ATP and preformed TNFα.

Stress also occurs during pregnancy as a response to factors impacting both the mother and fetus. In rats, stress induced by movement restriction has been observed to decrease mRNA levels as well as placental 11β-HSD2 activity but has a small or zero effect (depending on the study) on 11β-HSD1 mRNA levels [64, 65]. In the mothers, stress caused by food restriction leads to high levels of corticosterone and reduced levels of 11β-HSD2 mRNA expression at the placenta. This could affect the number of active GCs that are transferred from the mother to the fetuses, which would induce changes in their neurodevelopment [65].

Administration of the synthetic GC dexamethasone (DEX) in pregnant mammals induces neuroinflammation, which impacts the ontogeny of neurons and glia in the offspring [41, 70]. This synthetic glucocorticoid can cross the placental barrier, but it is not inactivated by 11β-HSD2, which could affect neuronal and glial maturation, as well as myelin synthesis, macrogliogenesis, and other processes in brain development [64, 71]. Furthermore, DEX modifies programmed and regulated glucocorticoid secretion and brain plasticity [41].

Diseases of different etiopathologies, such as depression [54, 72], schizophrenia [73], asthma [61, 74], preeclampsia [75], and Alzheimer's and Parkinson's disease [72, 76], have been linked to chronic GC release, which could enhance

GC-enhanced inflammation. GCs also have many applications in daily life. They are usually used as anti-inflammatory agents [54, 61], immunosuppressants, and in chemotherapy [54, 60]. The use of GCs as antenatal treatment is directed to reduce or prevent respiratory distress syndrome in premature fetuses. The direct correlation of an early increase in GC levels during development and adverse behavioral outcomes has been extensively described, including hypertension, gestational diabetes, autism, depression, and schizophrenia [77–80], and can be transmitted epigenetically [81]. The studies in humans are also supported by results obtained in experimental animals, including mice [41, 70, 82], rats [83–86], sheep [87, 88], and monkeys [89, 90]. In addition, the stress-induced changes in neuroanatomy are specific to brain region and sex [91, 92].

Elevated levels of GCs increase CRH levels, which in turn induce blood levels of ACTH [93] and the degranulation of mast cells [71]. While chronic stress increases GC levels and promotes the activation of NLRP3 in microglia [94, 95], astrocytes [96], and oligodendrocytes [41], it promotes the activation of NLRP1 in neurons [97]. Studies show a direct association between antenatal treatment with GCs and depression-like symptoms in offspring [83–85], inflammation [41], and/or changes in the hippocampus that have been associated with depression-like symptoms in adults [70, 82, 84, 86–90]. Examples of the relationship between neuroinflammation induced at prenatal stages and changes in behavior have been linked to toxic levels of lead [98]. Additionally, gossypol, a compound primarily found in the cotton plant, reduces neurogenesis by targeting the proliferation and differentiation of neuronal stem/progenitor cells, cognitive functions, and neuroinflammation [99].

4. Mast cells, microglia, and inflammation

In the brain, mast cells reside in vascularized regions, including the meninges, area postrema, choroid plexus, and the parenchyma of the thalamic-hypothalamic region [100]. They are characterized by granules loaded with proinflammatory molecules such as biogenic amines (histamines, serotonin), cytokines (e.g., IL1 to IL6 and TNFα), enzymes (e.g., phospholipases, tryptase), lipid metabolites (e.g., prostaglandins, leukotrienes), ATP, and growth factors, among others [18, 101–104]. Despite all these possibilities, it should be made clear that not all mast cells produce or maintain all these substances; rather, they depend on the environment and other conditions [103]. Furthermore, if a longer-lasting action is required, they produce de novo and release proinflammatory mediators [101]. Compared to other cell types in the CNS, the number of mast cells under regular conditions is low, but their ability to accumulate inflammatory effectors generates rapid responses to stress (mediated by CRH). The high content of inflammatory effectors and location (associated with the blood-brain barrier and leptomeninges) enables the mast cell degranulation response to be fast, amplified, and prolonged [101], which has been associated with different brain disorders [105].

In mammals, microglia develop in the embryonic sac, and as primitive macrophages, they enter the developing brain, colonizing the CNS parenchyma, where they mature into microglia [17, 106]. Microglia are a population distinct from mononuclear phagocytes, characterized by fulfilling multiple functions in the CNS. Their main function is the surveillance and protection of the nervous system, like macrophages, but they have other secondary functions such as maintaining homeostasis, tissue regeneration, removal of cellular debris, synaptogenesis, and production of trophic factors, among others. All this has led to the consideration of microglia as an important cell type within the CNS [17, 107, 108] in adults and during CNS development.

In response to a proinflammatory environment generated by the degranulation of mast cells, microglia move from their homeostatic state to a responding state, inducing changes in their phenotype and triggering motility toward the inflammatory signal (induced by ATP and/or TNFα in the extracellular milieu). Activating the inflammasome present in the microglia facilitates the inflammatory response [17, 107, 108], and this has been observed to be implicated in conditions like schizophrenia, major depressive disorder, anxiety, and autism spectrum disorder [109].

Astrocytes are a type of glial cell that play an important role in the regulation, maintenance, and promotion of neuronal synapses. They secrete soluble factors that target pre- and postsynaptic neurons, such as glutamate and L/D-serine, and can recycle neurotransmitters through transporters [16, 110]. This close relationship between neurons and astrocytes during the synapse led to the concept of "tripartite synapse." Increased levels of extracellular glutamate have been associated with depression in patients suffering from major depression and animal models of depression [110].

5. Connexons, pannexons, and neuroinflammation

Connexin-based gap junctions are constituted by clusters of intracellular channels that connect the cytoplasm of two contacting cells [50, 111]. The most studied gap junction channels are formed by two hemichannels, or connexons, which in turn are formed by six protein subunits called connexins. Most hemichannels are permeable to different ions and small molecules, many of them important for the maintenance of the inflammatory process and the assembly of the inflammasome, enabling the influx of Ca^{2+} and the efflux of glutamate and ATP [112, 113].

Pannexins present a similar membrane topology to connexins and form hemichannels called pannexons. The latter are constituted by seven pannexin protein subunits, which facilitate the release of ATP to the extracellular milieu [114, 115]. Recently, it has been reported that high levels of intracellular Ca^{2+} activate protease caspase-3 that cleaves the C-terminal domains of the pannexon. This increases the radius of the pannexon's pore, allowing for the influx of Ca^{2+} and maintaining permeability to ATP [116]. This function, related to the influx of Ca^{2+} and efflux of ATP (both of which are central in the inflammasome's activation and autocrine/paracrine inflammatory signaling), makes connexin and pannexin hemichannels potential molecular targets for interrupting stress-induced neuroinflammatory processes. Pannexins have also been reported to form gap junction channels [117], but their possible role in neuroinflammation remains elusive.

Accordingly, stress increases the activity of connexons, pannexons, and P2X7Rs in different brain cells [41, 69]. In adult male mice, chronic stress increases the activity of connexin43 hemichannels in microglia and astrocytes, as well as that of pannexin1 hemichannels in microglia, astrocytes, and neurons [69]. For example, newborn offspring of mice stressed with DEX during gestation show increased levels of connexin47, pannexin1, and P2X7R in oligodendrocytes that are maintained for several weeks, as well as an activation of the oligodendrocyte inflammasome [41]. Microglia activation has also been observed in the offspring of stressed pregnant rats, which could contribute to behavioral changes observed in adults with depression [118]. The offspring of mothers subjected to acute restraint stress show an increase in the activity of both connexin43 and pannexin1 hemichannels in astrocytes, which is further increased by chronic stress. After acute and chronic stress, pannexin1 hemichannel activity occurs in microglia and neurons.

Inhibiting glutamate NMDA/P2X7Rs can reduce chronic stress-induced hemichannel activity, whereas blocking connexin43 and pannexin1 hemichannels would fully reduce ATP and glutamate release, as observed in hippocampal slices from stressed mice. Releasing gliotransmitters through hemichannels has been proposed to participate in the pathogenesis of stress-associated psychiatric disorders [69]. Moreover, the induction of depression through chronic restraint stress and chronic unpredictable mild stress in rats has also been linked to the activation of connexin43 hemichannels and the release of glutamate and ATP [110].

Similarly, emotional or physical neglect due to abandonment is a clear source of stress in the early life of an infant. This type of stressor has been shown to be directly implicated in psychological symptoms such as inclination toward impulsive behavior, anxiety, depression, and others [119]. Dysregulation of astrocytic connexins has been identified in maternal isolation animal models that mimic early life stress [120]. A recent study showed that oligodendrocyte precursor cells have a prominent role in modulating brain function and diseases through the paracrine regulation of astrocyte development. This could provide a possible explanation for previous findings, where the altered morphology of astrocytes in patients with mental disorders was observed to be associated with a reduced number of oligodendroglial lineage cells [119]. Clearly, in adults, neuroinflammation is present in models of social defeat stress [121], but further studies are required to validate the influence of different types of stress, such as psychosocial stress and unpredictable mild stress or social defeat paradigms, on the intensity and duration of neuroinflammation and CNS cytoarchitecture at different ages. Interestingly, chronic unpredictable mild stress has been associated with low expression of NLRP3 [122], strongly suggesting that reduced neuroinflammation renders protection.

Hemichannels belong to the family of large-pore channels, which includes transient receptor potential (TRP) channels, Piezo channels, CAHLM channels, and P2X receptors, all of which are nonselective channels permeable to small molecules and cations like Ca^{2+}. Some of them, like connexins, truncated pannexin1 hemichannels, and CAHLM1 channels, are expressed in most cell types, sharing structural and pharmacological sensitivity [123]. To show their involvement in any brain disease, it is, thus, critical to demonstrate their selectivity.

The compound D4 ((R)-2-(4-chlorophenyl)-2-oxo-1-phenylethyl quinolone-2-carboxylate, MW: 401.85 g/mol) inhibits the passage of molecules through connexin hemichannels, functioning as a blocker. This small organic molecule does not block connexin gap junction channels [124], CAHLM1 channels [125], or P2X7Rs [126]. Initial studies showed the ability to reduce atrophy in pathological muscle dysfunctions [127], as well as decrease neuroinflammation in temporal lobe epilepsy [128]. D4 has also been shown to inhibit stress-mediated astrogliosis and induce restoration of neural activity at the brain level in adult mice with depression-like symptoms [126]. Likewise, the compounds TAT-Cx43L2 and cacotheline have been studied and linked to blocking connexin43 hemichannels after the induction of depression through chronic stress. Subcutaneous cacotheline has been shown to have antidepressant effects by specifically preventing connexin43 hemichannel activity in a similar fashion as D4 [110]. Other approaches to inhibiting hemichannels include peptides like TAT-Gap 19, which exert an anticonvulsant effect in rodents [129] and protect from cerebral ischemia/reperfusion injury [130, 131]. Other small organic molecules, such as CVB2-61, a phenolic diaryl ether, and a curcuminoid analog, have been proposed to inhibit connexin hemichannels [132] and, therefore, might be useful toward reducing neuroinflammation in several brain diseases. The importance of neuroinflammation in the development of epilepsy has also been proposed using other drugs such as lacosamide and amlexanox [133, 134], supporting the concept that neuroinflammation plays a relevant role in epilepsy.

One of the most interesting compounds that has been shown to block connexin hemichannels in animal and cell models is Tonabersat, which reduces the effects of damage in the retina of rats [135, 136] and the inhibition of ATP release through connexin43 in cell cultures [136, 137]. Tonabersat is being tested in clinical trials for other uses (migraines, diabetic macular edema, and long COVID) [138], which can facilitate its use in the future for neuroinflammation in human patients. A different approach could be the use of a polypharmacology agent like boldine, which blocks connexin and pannexin hemichannels and P2X7Rs [125, 127, 139].

With all the background presented, a neuroinflammatory process in offspring, due to an increase in GCs in the mother during the gestational period, can be expected to have effects that are observed at birth and remain until adulthood. The decrease or increase in dendritic arborization and density, as well as the chronic activation of macroglia, microglia, and the inflammasome, would produce a neuroinflammatory environment in relevant brain areas, which would be reflected in the appearance of symptoms like anxiety disorders or depression in adult mice. This effect could be diminished by blocking connexin hemichannels with the use of the anti-inflammatory molecule D4. Reducing these complex disorders to a hemichannel-inflammation axis risks oversimplification. However, it seems to offer an alternative that could be tested in humans because current treatments focusing on neuronal targets appear poorly effective according to a network meta-analysis study [140].

6. Epigenetic changes induced by stress

Epigenetics refers to short- and long-term gene expression variations that are caused by non-DNA-encoded mechanisms. These changes are hereditary and include the methylation of cytosine bases, acetylation, and the methylation of histones and nonhistone proteins, as well as changes in noncoding RNA expression, chromatin remodeling, and RNA modification [141, 142].

Conditions such as autism spectrum disorder, depression, anxiety disorders, post-traumatic stress disorder, and schizophrenia present epigenetic modification [3, 142–145]. Chronic stress is known to induce persistent changes in global DNA methylation and gene expression in different brain areas [146]. Several enzymes can reverse epigenetic changes, with key players including histone deacetylases and DNA methyltransferases. Histone deacetylases remove acetyl groups from histones, while DNA methyltransferases remove methyl groups from DNA, effectively undoing these epigenetic modifications. Research on epigenetic therapies suggests strong evidence for normal gene expression restoration linked to inhibitors and modulators of the activity of enzymes involved in epigenetic modifications, like DNA methylation and histone acetylation. This allows for the reversal of abnormal epigenetic patterns and can be used to treat diseases where epigenetic changes are implicated. Pharmacological inhibitors of DNA methylation, such as azacitidine and decitabine, were developed to reverse epigenetic changes *via* DNA methyltransferase inhibition. It has been proposed that some antidepressant drugs may exert direct epigenetic effects. For instance, tricyclic antidepressants amitriptyline and imipramine have been shown to reduce promoter DNA methylation in rat primary astrocytes, presumably by reducing DNA methyltransferase 1 activity [147, 148].

The use of epigenetic drugs can also help to alleviate the symptoms of some neurodegenerative diseases or neurodevelopmental conditions. LSD1, a selective inhibitor of H3K4me2 demethylase, has been shown to reverse some of the most common behaviors of an autistic mouse model, such as social deficits and repetitive movements [149]. Similarly, the use of several drugs used as mood stabilizers, antidepressants, and/or for the treatment of epilepsy, such as valproate, lithium chloride, and clozapine, among others, induces changes in the different histone acetylases in the brain [150]. This network suggests the idea that a combination of drugs targeting connexin and pannexin hemichannels, in conjunction with epigenetic drugs, could generate synergistic effects and favor the recovery of DNA in a condition not associated with behavioral diseases.

7. Concluding remarks

In the quest to find molecular targets that reduce or block neuroinflammation, connexin hemichannels expressed by glial cells appear to be good candidates. Given that the hemichannels found in the cell membrane are of easy access, they appear to be a good pharmacological target to achieve this goal. In fact, several pharmacological approaches have been tested and have revealed relevant protective action in animal models of human diseases. They include the small organic molecule D4, TAT-Gap 19 peptide, Tonabersat, TAT-CX43L2, cacotheline, and boldine, which could be part of a new generation of anti-inflammatory drugs.

As seen in this chapter, a large body of studies indicates that homeostatic disorders in the developing CNS due to chronic stress during the prenatal stages of the mother or the early life of the offspring can lead to a neuroinflammatory environment that favors changes, some or all of which involve several steps of brain ontogeny (cell migration, proliferation, maturation, and differentiation) being part of the balanced process for the normal development of the CNS. Any change could lead to the first events that, sooner or later, can result in neuropsychiatric diseases or conditions.

Different levels or intensities of stress are commonplace in our modern days. It is relevant today more than ever to assess their effects on the development and ontogeny of the CNS and, consequently, on the development and ontogeny of neuroinflammation that can result in neuropsychiatric disorders or conditions. Establishing treatments that reduce or even block neuroinflammation by using hemichannel blockers and/or epigenetic drugs could be a promising start toward reducing the negative effects of neuroinflammation in the ontogeny and development of the CNS. Further studies are required to understand the relative involvement of neuroinflammation in behavioral diseases, as compared to other working hypotheses, such as dysregulation of dopamine in certain brain regions in the development and maintenance of depressive symptoms [151].

Although the development of pharmacological tools has provided novel interpretations on the etiopathogenesis of diverse brain malfunctions in different chronic diseases, the development of conditional connexin and pannexin cell-specific knockouts will provide valuable information to strengthen the interpretation of different findings in this area of research. Accordingly, Cx43 KO in microglia has recently supported the role of connexin hemichannels in neuroinflammation and progression of Alzheimer's disease [152].

DOI: http://dx.doi.org/10.5772/intechopen.1012583

Acknowledgements

This work was partially supported by the Agencia Nacional de Investigación y Desarrollo (ANID) grant 1231523 (to JCS) and the Doctoral thesis support fellowship at Valparaíso University (to FJO). The primary proposal was presented by FJO to partially fulfill the requirements for a Doctor of Science degree with a specialization in Neuroscience at the University of Valparaiso.

Conflicts of interest

The authors declare no conflict of interest.

Author details

Francisco J. Ocaranza and Juan C. Sáez*
Neuroscience Institute, Interdisciplinary Neuroscience Center of Valparaíso, University of Valparaíso, Chile

*Address all correspondence to: juancarlos.saez@uv.cl

References

[1] Robinson R, Lähdepuro A, Tuovinen S, et al. Maternal hypertensive pregnancy disorders and mental and behavioral disorders in the offspring: A review. Current Hypertension Reports. 2021;**23**:30. DOI: 10.1007/s11906-021-01141-w

[2] Kelly SJ, Day N, Streissguth AP. Effects of prenatal alcohol exposure on social behavior in humans and other species. Neurotoxicology and Teratology. 2000;**22**:143-149. DOI: 10.1016/S0892-0362(99)00073-2

[3] Cattane N, Richetto J, Cattaneo A. Prenatal exposure to environmental insults and enhanced risk of developing schizophrenia and autism spectrum disorder: Focus on biological pathways and epigenetic mechanisms. Neuroscience & Biobehavioral Reviews. 2020;**117**:253-278. DOI: 10.1016/j.neubiorev.2018.07.001

[4] Shin SH, Kim YK. Early life stress, neuroinflammation, and psychiatric illness of adulthood. Advances in Experimental Medicine and Biology. 2023;**1411**:105-134. DOI: 10.1007/978-981-19-7376-5_6

[5] Oronsky B, Caroen S, Reid T. What exactly is inflammation (and what is it not?). International Journal of Molecular Sciences. 2022;**23**:14905. DOI: 10.3390/ijms232314905

[6] Rea K, Dinan TG, Cryan JF. The microbiome: A key regulator of stress and neuroinflammation. Neurobiology of Stress. 2016;**4**:23-33. DOI: 10.1016/j.ynstr.2016.03.001

[7] Penisson M, Ladewig J, Belvindrah R, et al. Genes and mechanisms involved in the generation and amplification of basal radial glial cells. Frontiers in Cellular Neuroscience. 2019;**13**:1-21. DOI: 10.3389/fncel.2019.00381

[8] Zhang J, Tabassum S, Jiang J, et al. Optimized Golgi-Cox staining validated in the hippocampus of spared nerve injury mouse model. Frontiers in Neuroanatomy. 2020;**14**:1-10. DOI: 10.3389/fnana.2020.585513

[9] Kissinger R. Macrophage. NIAID Visual & Medical Arts; 2024. Available from: https://bioart.niaid.nih.gov/bioart/310 [Accessed: May 11, 2025]

[10] Kissinger R. Astrocyte. NIAID Visual & Medical Arts; 2024. Available from: https://bioart.niaid.nih.gov/bioart/40 [Accessed: May 11, 2025]

[11] Kissinger R. Immature Organoid Brush. NIAID Visual & Medical Arts; 2024. Available from: https://bioart.niaid.nih.gov/bioart/251 [Accessed: May 11, 2025]

[12] Reemst K, Noctor SC, Lucassen PJ, et al. The indispensable roles of microglia and astrocytes during brain development. Frontiers in Human Neuroscience. 2016;**10**:1-28

[13] Nishiyama A, Shimizu T, Sherafat A, et al. Life-long oligodendrocyte development and plasticity. Seminars in Cell & Developmental Biology. 2021;**116**:25-37. DOI: 10.1016/j.semcdb.2021.02.004

[14] Li X, Liu G, Yang L, et al. Decoding cortical glial cell development. Neuroscience Bulletin. 2021;**37**:440-460. DOI: 10.1007/s12264-021-00640-9

[15] Vivi E, Di Benedetto B. Brain stars take the lead during critical periods of early postnatal brain development:

Relevance of astrocytes in health and mental disorders. Molecular Psychiatry. 2024;**29**:2821-2833. DOI: 10.1038/s41380-024-02534-4

[16] Farhy-Tselnicker I, Allen NJ. Astrocytes, neurons, synapses: A tripartite view on cortical circuit development. Neural Development. 2018;**13**:7-19

[17] Nayak D, Roth TL, McGavern DB. Microglia development and function. Annual Review of Immunology. 2014;**32**:367-402. DOI: 10.1146/annurev-immunol-032713-120240

[18] St. John AL, APS R, Ginhoux F. New perspectives on the origins and heterogeneity of mast cells. Nature Reviews Immunology. 2023;**23**:55-68. DOI: 10.1038/s41577-022-00731-2

[19] Stagni F, Giacomini A, Guidi S, et al. Timing of therapies for down syndrome: The sooner, the better. Frontiers in Behavioral Neuroscience. 2015;**9**:1-18

[20] Chilton J. Mast Cell. SciDrawIo; 2024. DOI: 10.5281/zenodo.14284999

[21] He F. Oligodendrocyte Progenitor Cell. SciDrawIo; 2023. DOI: 10.5281/zenodo.7787767

[22] Chilton J. Astrocyte. SciDrawIo; 2020. DOI: 10.5281/zenodo.3926048

[23] Chilton J. Microglia Reactive. SciDrawIo; 2020. DOI: 10.5281/zenodo.3926211

[24] Chilton J. Neuron. SciDrawIo; 2020. DOI: 10.5281/zenodo.3926009

[25] Maras PM, Molet J, Chen Y, et al. Preferential loss of dorsal-hippocampus synapses underlies memory impairments provoked by short, multimodal stress. Molecular Psychiatry. 2014;**19**:811-822. DOI: 10.1038/mp.2014.12

[26] Chenani A, Weston G, Ulivi AF, et al. Repeated stress exposure leads to structural synaptic instability prior to disorganization of hippocampal coding and impairments in learning. Translational Psychiatry. 2022;**12**:381. DOI: 10.1038/s41398-022-02107-5

[27] Aguirre A, Maturana CJ, Harcha PA, et al. Possible involvement of TLRs and hemichannels in stress-induced CNS dysfunction via mastocytes, and glia activation. Mediators of Inflammation. 2013;**2013**:1-17. DOI: 10.1155/2013/893521

[28] Sun SC. The non-canonical NF-κB pathway in immunity and inflammation. Nature Reviews Immunology. 2017;**17**:545-558. DOI: 10.1038/nri.2017.52

[29] Madrigal J. The increase in TNF-α levels is implicated in NF-κB activation and inducible nitric oxide synthase expression in brain cortex after immobilization stress. Neuropsychopharmacology. 2002;**26**:155-163. DOI: 10.1016/S0893-133X(01)00292-5

[30] Sorrells SF, Caso JR, Munhoz CD, et al. The stressed CNS: When glucocorticoids aggravate inflammation. Neuron. 2009;**64**:33-39. DOI: 10.1016/j.neuron.2009.09.032

[31] Franchi L, Eigenbrod T, Núñez G. Cutting edge: TNF-α mediates sensitization to ATP and silica via the NLRP3 inflammasome in the absence of microbial stimulation. The Journal of Immunology. 2009;**183**:792-796. DOI: 10.4049/jimmunol.0900173

[32] Petrilli V, Papin S, Tschopp J. The inflammasome. Current Biology. 2005;**15**:R581. DOI: 10.1016/j.cub.2005.07.049

[33] Sandhu JK, Kulka M. Decoding mast cell-microglia communication in

neurodegenerative diseases. International Journal of Molecular Sciences. 2021;**22**:1-22. DOI: 10.3390/ijms22031093

[34] Kissinger R. Inflammasome. NIAID Visual & Medical Arts; 2024. Available from: https://bioart.niaid.nih.gov/bioart/255 [Accessed: May 11, 2025]

[35] Kissinger R. Receptor. NIAID Visual & Medical Arts; 2024. Available from: https://bioart.niaid.nih.gov/bioart/429 [Accessed: May 11, 2025]

[36] Kissinger R. DNA. NIAID Visual & Medical Arts; 2024. Available from: https://bioart.niaid.nih.gov/bioart/123 [Accessed: May 11, 2025]

[37] Servier Medical Art. Membrane (Yellow-Orange). Servier Medical Art. 2025. Available from: https://bioicons.com/?query=membrane-2d-yelloworange%20 [Accessed: May 11, 2025]

[38] Servier Medical Art. Channel (Yellow). Servier Medical Art. 2025. Available from: https://smart.servier.com/smart_image/smart-yellow-channel-tubes-overview/ [Accessed: May 11, 2025]

[39] Servier Medical Art. Channel (Red). Servier Medical Art. 2025. Available from: https://smart.servier.com/smart_image/smart-red-channel-overview/ [Accessed: May 11, 2025]

[40] Servier Medical Art. Channel (Blue Sky). Servier Medical Art. 2025. Available from: https://smart.servier.com/smart_image/blue-sky-channels/ [Accessed: May 11, 2025]

[41] Maturana CJ, Aguirre A, Sáez JC. High glucocorticoid levels during gestation activate the inflammasome in hippocampal oligodendrocytes of the offspring. Developmental Neurobiology. 2017;**77**:625-642. DOI: 10.1002/dneu.22409

[42] Chen R, Yin C, Fang J, et al. The NLRP3 inflammasome: An emerging therapeutic target for chronic pain. Journal of Neuroinflammation. 2021;**18**. DOI: 10.1186/s12974-021-02131-0

[43] Grol MW, Zelner I, Dixon SJ. P2X 7-mediated calcium influx triggers a sustained, PI3K-dependent increase in metabolic acid production by osteoblast-like cells. American Journal of Physiology-Endocrinology and Metabolism. 2012;**302**:561-575. DOI: 10.1152/ajpendo.00209.2011.-The

[44] Liang X, Samways DSK, Wolf K, et al. Quantifying Ca^{2+} current and permeability in ATP-gated P2X7 receptors. Journal of Biological Chemistry. 2015;**290**:7930-7942. DOI: 10.1074/jbc.M114.627810

[45] Cotrina ML, Lin JH-C, Alves-Rodrigues A, et al. Connexins regulate calcium signaling by controlling ATP release. Proceedings of the National Academy of Sciences. 1998;**95**:15735-15740. DOI: 10.1073/pnas.95.26.15735

[46] Arcuino G, Lin JH-C, Takano T, et al. Intercellular calcium signaling mediated by point-source burst release of ATP. Proceedings of the National Academy of Sciences. 2002;**99**:9840-9845. DOI: 10.1073/pnas.152588599

[47] Gustin A, Kirchmeyer M, Koncina E, et al. NLRP3 inflammasome is expressed and functional in mouse brain microglia but not in astrocytes. PLoS One. 2015;**10**:e0130624. DOI: 10.1371/journal.pone.0130624

[48] Albalawi F, Lu W, Beckel JM, et al. The P2X7 receptor primes IL-1β and the NLRP3 inflammasome in astrocytes exposed to mechanical strain. Frontiers

in Cellular Neuroscience. 2017;**11**:1-14. DOI: 10.3389/fncel.2017.00227

[49] Zhang X, Wang R, Hu D, et al. Oligodendroglial glycolytic stress triggers inflammasome activation and neuropathology in Alzheimer's disease. Science Advances. 2020;**6**:eabb8680. DOI: 10.1126/sciadv.abb8680

[50] Li D-X, Wang C-N, Wang Y, et al. NLRP3 inflammasome-dependent pyroptosis and apoptosis in hippocampus neurons mediates depressive-like behavior in diabetic mice. Behavioural Brain Research. 2020;**391**:112684. DOI: 10.1016/j.bbr.2020.112684

[51] Mychasiuk R, Gibb R, Kolb B. Prenatal stress alters dendritic morphology and synaptic connectivity in the prefrontal cortex and hippocampus of developing offspring. Synapse. 2012;**66**:308-314. DOI: 10.1002/syn.21512

[52] Radley JJ, Rocher AB, Miller M, et al. Repeated stress induces dendritic spine loss in the rat medial prefrontal cortex. Cerebral Cortex. 2006;**16**:313-320. DOI: 10.1093/cercor/bhi104

[53] Liston C, Miller MM, Goldwater DS, et al. Stress-induced alterations in prefrontal cortical dendritic morphology predict selective impairments in perceptual attentional set-shifting. Journal of Neuroscience. 2006;**26**:7870-7874. DOI: 10.1523/JNEUROSCI.1184-06.2006

[54] Cain DW, Cidlowski JA. Immune regulation by glucocorticoids. Nature Reviews Immunology. 2017;**17**:233-247. DOI: 10.1038/nri.2017.1

[55] Habib KE, Gold PW, Chrousos GP. Neuroendocrinology of stress. Endocrinology and Metabolism Clinics of North America. 2001;**30**:695-728. DOI: 10.1016/S0889-8529(05)70208-5

[56] Kemeny ME. The psychobiology of stress. Current Directions in Psychological Science. 2003;**12**:124-129. DOI: 10.1111/1467-8721.01246

[57] Chan S, Debono M. Replication of cortisol circadian rhythm: New advances in hydrocortisone replacement therapy. Therapeutic Advances in Endocrinology and Metabolism. 2010;**1**:129-138. DOI: 10.1177/2042018810380214

[58] Dickmeis T. Glucocorticoids and the circadian clock. Journal of Endocrinology. 2009;**200**:3-22. DOI: 10.1677/JOE-08-0415

[59] Liddle GW. Analysis of circadian rhythms in human adrenocortical secretory activity. Archives of Internal Medicine. 1966;**117**:739-743

[60] Smith LK, Cidlowski JA. Glucocorticoid-induced apoptosis of healthy and malignant lymphocytes. Progress in Brain Research. 2010;**182**:1-30. DOI: 10.1016/s0079-6123(10)82001-1

[61] Adcock IM, Mumby S. Glucocorticoids. In: Handbook of Experimental Pharmacology. Vol. 237. New York: Springer, LLC; 2016. pp. 171-196. DOI: 10.1007/164_2016_98

[62] Galon J, Franchimont D, Hiroi N, et al. Gene profiling reveals unknown enhancing and suppressive actions of glucocorticoids on immune cells. The FASEB Journal. 2002;**16**:61-71. DOI: 10.1096/fj.01-0245com

[63] Seckl JR. 11β-hydroxysteroid dehydrogenases: Changing glucocorticoid action. Current Opinion in Pharmacology. 2004;**4**:597-602. DOI: 10.1016/j.coph.2004.09.001

[64] Mairesse J, Lesage J, Breton C, et al. Maternal stress alters endocrine function of the feto-placental unit in

rats. American Journal of Physiology-Endocrinology and Metabolism. 2007;**292**:E1526-E1533. DOI: 10.1152/ajpendo.00574.2006

[65] Jensen Peña C, Monk C, Champagne FA. Epigenetic effects of prenatal stress on 11β-hydroxysteroid dehydrogenase-2 in the placenta and fetal brain. PLoS One. 2012;**7**:e39791. DOI: 10.1371/journal.pone.0039791

[66] Necela BM, Cidlowski JA. Mechanisms of glucocorticoid receptor action in noninflammatory and inflammatory cells. Proceedings of the American Thoracic Society. 2004;**1**:239-246. DOI: 10.1513/pats.200402-005MS

[67] Sorrells SF, Sapolsky RM. An inflammatory review of glucocorticoid actions in the CNS. Brain, Behavior, and Immunity. 2007;**21**:259-272. DOI: 10.1016/j.bbi.2006.11.006

[68] Căruntu C, Boda D, Musat S, et al. Stress-induced mast cell activation in glabrous and hairy skin. Mediators of Inflammation. 2014;**2014**:1-9. DOI: 10.1155/2014/105950

[69] Orellana JA, Moraga-Amaro R, Díaz-Galarce R, et al. Restraint stress increases hemichannel activity in hippocampal glial cells and neurons. Frontiers in Cellular Neuroscience. 2015;**9**:1-12. DOI: 10.3389/fncel.2015.00102

[70] Noorlander CW, Tijsseling D, Hessel EVS, et al. Antenatal glucocorticoid treatment affects hippocampal development in mice. PLoS One. 2014;**9**:e85671. DOI: 10.1371/journal.pone.0085671

[71] Esposito P, Chandler N, Kandere K, et al. Corticotropin-releasing hormone and brain mast cells regulate blood-brain-barrier permeability induced by acute stress. The Journal of Pharmacology and Experimental Therapeutics. 2002;**303**:1061-1066. DOI: 10.1124/jpet.102.038497

[72] Swaab DF, Bao AM, Lucassen PJ. The stress system in the human brain in depression and neurodegeneration. Ageing Research Reviews. 2005;**4**:141-194. DOI: 10.1016/j.arr.2005.03.003

[73] Ph.D. J. Glucocorticoid hormones and early brain development in schizophrenia. Neuropsychopharmacology. 2002;**27**:309-318. DOI: 10.1016/S0893-133X(01)00396-7

[74] Panettieri RA, Schaafsma D, Amrani Y, et al. Non-genomic effects of glucocorticoids: An updated view. Trends in Pharmacological Sciences. 2019;**40**:38-49. DOI: 10.1016/j.tips.2018.11.002

[75] Vianna P, Bauer ME, Dornfeld D, et al. Distress conditions during pregnancy may lead to pre-eclampsia by increasing cortisol levels and altering lymphocyte sensitivity to glucocorticoids. Medical Hypotheses. 2011;**77**:188-191. DOI: 10.1016/j.mehy.2011.04.007

[76] Kline SA, Mega MS. Stress-induced neurodegeneration: The potential for coping as neuroprotective therapy. American Journal of Alzheimer's Disease and Other Dementias. 2020;**35**:1-13. DOI: 10.1177/1533317520960873

[77] Kay VR, Rätsep MT, Figueiró-Filho EA, et al. Preeclampsia may influence offspring neuroanatomy and cognitive function: A role for placental growth factor. Biology of Reproduction. 2019;**101**:271-283. DOI: 10.1093/biolre/ioz095

[78] Rose'Meyer R. A review of the serotonin transporter and prenatal cortisol in the development of autism

spectrum disorders. Molecular Autism. 2013;**4**:37. DOI: 10.1186/2040-2392-4-37

[79] Welberg LAM, Seckl JR. Prenatal stress, glucocorticoids and the programming of the brain. Journal of Neuroendocrinology. 2001;**13**:113-128. DOI: 10.1111/j.1365-2826.2001.00601.x

[80] Harris A, Seckl J. Glucocorticoids, prenatal stress and the programming of disease. Hormones and Behavior. 2011;**59**:279-289. DOI: 10.1016/j.yhbeh.2010.06.007

[81] Oberlander TF, Weinberg J, Papsdorf M, et al. Prenatal exposure to maternal depression, neonatal methylation of human glucocorticoid receptor gene (NR3C1) and infant cortisol stress responses. Epigenetics. 2008;**3**:97-106. DOI: 10.4161/epi.3.2.6034

[82] Noorlander CW, Visser GHA, Ramakers GMJ, et al. Prenatal corticosteroid exposure affects hippocampal plasticity and reduces lifespan. Developmental Neurobiology. 2008;**68**:237-246. DOI: 10.1002/dneu.20583

[83] Vázquez DM, Neal CR, Patel PD, et al. Regulation of corticoid and serotonin receptor brain system following early life exposure of glucocorticoids: Long term implications for the neurobiology of mood. Psychoneuroendocrinology. 2012;**37**:421-437. DOI: 10.1016/j.psyneuen.2011.07.012

[84] Głombik K, Kukla-Bartoszek M, Curzytek K, et al. The effects of prenatal dexamethasone exposure on brain metabolic homeostasis in adulthood: Implications for depression. International Journal of Molecular Sciences. 2023;**24**:1156. DOI: 10.3390/ijms24021156

[85] Hiroi R, Carbone DL, Zuloaga DG, et al. Sex-dependent programming effects of prenatal glucocorticoid treatment on the developing serotonin system and stress-related behaviors in adulthood. Neuroscience. 2016;**320**:43-56. DOI: 10.1016/j.neuroscience.2016.01.055

[86] Huang C-C, Lin H-R, Liang Y-C, et al. Effects of neonatal corticosteroid treatment on hippocampal synaptic function. Pediatric Research. 2007;**62**:267-270. DOI: 10.1203/PDR.0b013e318123f744

[87] Huang W. Effect of corticosteroids on brain growth in fetal sheep. Obstetrics & Gynecology. 1999;**94**:213-218. DOI: 10.1016/S0029-7844(99)00265-3

[88] Huang WL, Harper CG, Evans SF, et al. Repeated prenatal corticosteroid administration delays astrocyte and capillary tight junction maturation in fetal sheep. International Journal of Developmental Neuroscience. 2001;**19**:487-493. DOI: 10.1016/S0736-5748(01)00035-1

[89] Uno H, Lohmiller L, Thieme C, et al. Brain damage induced by prenatal exposure to dexamethasone in fetal rhesus macaques. I. Hippocampus. Developmental Brain Research. 1990;**53**:157-167. DOI: 10.1016/0165-3806(90)90002-G

[90] Tauber SC, Schlumbohm C, Schilg L, et al. Intrauterine exposure to dexamethasone impairs proliferation but not neuronal differentiation in the dentate gyrus of newborn common marmoset monkeys. Brain Pathology. 2006;**16**:209-217. DOI: 10.1111/j.1750-3639.2006.00021.x

[91] Kolb B, Gibb R. Plasticity in the prefrontal cortex of adult rats. Frontiers in Cellular Neuroscience. 2015;**9**:1-11. DOI: 10.3389/fncel.2015.00015

[92] Arnsten AFT. Stress signalling pathways that impair prefrontal cortex

structure and function. Nature Reviews Neuroscience. 2009;**10**:410-422. DOI: 10.1038/nrn2648

[93] Tauchi M, Zhang R, D'Alessio DA, et al. Role of central glucagon-like peptide-1 in hypothalamo-pituitary-adrenocortical facilitation following chronic stress. Experimental Neurology. 2008;**210**:458-466. DOI: 10.1016/j.expneurol.2007.11.016

[94] Frank MG, Hershman SA, Weber MD, et al. Chronic exposure to exogenous glucocorticoids primes microglia to pro-inflammatory stimuli and induces NLRP3 mRNA in the hippocampus. Psychoneuroendocrinology. 2014;**40**:191-200. DOI: 10.1016/j.psyneuen.2013.11.006

[95] Bharti V, Tan H, Zhou H, et al. Txnip mediates glucocorticoid-activated NLRP3 inflammatory signaling in mouse microglia. Neurochemistry International. 2019;**131**:104564. DOI: 10.1016/j.neuint.2019.104564

[96] Yue N, Huang H, Zhu X, et al. Activation of P2X7 receptor and NLRP3 inflammasome assembly in hippocampal glial cells mediates chronic stress-induced depressive-like behaviors. Journal of Neuroinflammation. 2017;**14**:102. DOI: 10.1186/s12974-017-0865-y

[97] Zhang B, Zhang Y, Xu T, et al. Chronic dexamethasone treatment results in hippocampal neurons injury due to activate NLRP1 inflammasome in vitro. International Immunopharmacology. 2017;**49**:222-230. DOI: 10.1016/j.intimp.2017.05.039

[98] Cory-Slechta DA, Sobolewski M, Varma G, et al. Developmental lead and/or prenatal stress exposures followed by different types of behavioral experience result in the divergence of brain epigenetic profiles in a sex, brain region, and time-dependent manner: Implications for neurotoxicology. Current Opinion in Toxicology. 2017;**6**:60-70. DOI: 10.1016/j.cotox.2017.09.004

[99] Zhu X, Wu Y, Pan J, et al. Neuroinflammation induction and alteration of hippocampal neurogenesis in mice following developmental exposure to gossypol. International Journal of Neuropsychopharmacology. 2021;**24**:419-433. DOI: 10.1093/ijnp/pyaa093

[100] Harcha PA, Garcés P, Arredondo C, et al. Mast cell and astrocyte hemichannels and their role in Alzheimer's disease, ALS, and harmful stress conditions. International Journal of Molecular Sciences. 2021;**22**:1-19. DOI: 10.3390/ijms22041924

[101] Dong H, Zhang X, Qian Y. Mast cells and neuroinflammation. Medical Science Monitor Basic Research. 2014;**20**:200-206. DOI: 10.12659/MSMBR.893093

[102] Grootens J, Ungerstedt JS, Nilsson G, et al. Deciphering the differentiation trajectory from hematopoietic stem cells to mast cells. Blood Advances. 2018;**2**:2273-2281. DOI: 10.1182/bloodadvances.2018019539

[103] Galli SJ, Kalesnikoff J, Grimbaldeston MA, et al. Mast cells as "tunable" effector and immunoregulatory cells: Recent advances. Annual Review of Immunology. 2005;**23**:749-786. DOI: 10.1146/annurev.immunol.21.120601.141025

[104] Wang L, Sikora J, Hu L, et al. ATP release from mast cells by physical stimulation: A putative early step in activation of acupuncture points. Evidence-based Complementary and

Alternative Medicine. 2013;**2013**:1-7. DOI: 10.1155/2013/350949

[105] Huang X, Lan Z, Hu Z. Role and mechanisms of mast cells in brain disorders. Frontiers in Immunology. 2024;**15**:1445867. DOI: 10.3389/fimmu.2024.1445867

[106] McGrath KE, Frame JM, Palis J. Early hematopoiesis and macrophage development. Seminars in Immunology. 2015;**27**:379-387. DOI: 10.1016/j.smim.2016.03.013

[107] Bolós M, Perea JR, Avila J. Alzheimer's disease as an inflammatory disease. Biomolecular Concepts. 2017;**8**:37-43. DOI: 10.1515/bmc-2016-0029

[108] Paolicelli RC, Sierra A, Stevens B, et al. Microglia states and nomenclature: A field at its crossroads. Neuron. 2022;**110**:3458-3483. DOI: 10.1016/j.neuron.2022.10.020

[109] Frick LR, Williams K, Pittenger C. Microglial dysregulation in psychiatric disease. Clinical & Developmental Immunology. 2013;**2013**:1-10. DOI: 10.1155/2013/608654

[110] Duarte Y, Quintana-Donoso D, Moraga-Amaro R, et al. The role of astrocytes in depression, its prevention, and treatment by targeting astroglial gliotransmitter release. Proceedings of the National Academy of Sciences. 2024;**121**:1-12. DOI: 10.1073/pnas.2307953121

[111] Sáez JC, Brañes MC, Corvalán LA, et al. Gap junctions in cells of the immune system: Structure, regulation and possible functional roles. Brazilian Journal of Medical and Biological Research. 2000;**33**:447-455. DOI: 10.1590/S0100-879X2000000400011

[112] Schalper KA, Sánchez HA, Lee SC, et al. Connexin 43 hemichannels mediate the Ca^{2+} influx induced by extracellular alkalinization. American Journal of Physiology-Cell Physiology. 2010;**299**:C1504-C1515. DOI: 10.1152/ajpcell.00015.2010

[113] Abudara V, Retamal MA, Del Rio R, et al. Synaptic functions of hemichannels and pannexons: A double-edged sword. Frontiers in Molecular Neuroscience. 2018;**11**:1-24. DOI: 10.3389/fnmol.2018.00435

[114] Adamson SE, Leitinger N. The role of pannexin1 in the induction and resolution of inflammation. FEBS Letters. 2014;**588**:1416-1422. DOI: 10.1016/j.febslet.2014.03.009

[115] Yi WJ, Kim TS. Melatonin protects mice against stress-induced inflammation through enhancement of M2 macrophage polarization. International Immunopharmacology. 2017;**48**:146-158. DOI: 10.1016/j.intimp.2017.05.006

[116] Salgado M, Márquez-Miranda V, Ferrada L, et al. Ca^{2+} permeation through C-terminal cleaved, but not full-length human Pannexin1 hemichannels, mediates cell death. Proceedings of the National Academy of Sciences. 2024;**121**:1-10. DOI: 10.1073/pnas.2405468121

[117] Palacios-Prado N, Soto PA, López X, et al. Endogenous pannexin1 channels form functional intercellular cell–cell channels with characteristic voltage-dependent properties. Proceedings of the National Academy of Sciences. 2022;**119**:1-11. DOI: 10.1073/pnas.2202104119

[118] Ślusarczyk J, Trojan E, Głombik K, et al. Prenatal stress is a vulnerability factor for altered morphology and biological activity of microglia cells. Frontiers in Cellular Neuroscience.

2015;**9**:1-14. DOI: 10.3389/fncel.2015.00082

[119] Wang Y, Su Y, Yu G, et al. Reduced oligodendrocyte precursor cell impairs astrocytic development in early life stress. Advanced Science. 2021;**8**:2101181. DOI: 10.1002/advs.202101181

[120] Çalışkan G, Müller A, Albrecht A. Long-term impact of early-life stress on hippocampal plasticity: Spotlight on astrocytes. International Journal of Molecular Sciences. 2020;**21**:1-19. DOI: 10.3390/ijms21144999

[121] Bravo-Tobar ID, Fernández P, Sáez JC, et al. Long-term effects of stress resilience: Hippocampal neuroinflammation and behavioral approach in male rats. Journal of Neuroscience Research. 2021;**99**:2493-2510. DOI: 10.1002/jnr.24902

[122] Yang Y, Xing M-J, Li Y, et al. Reduced NLRP3 inflammasome expression in the brain is associated with stress resilience. Psychoneuroendocrinology. 2021;**128**:105211. DOI: 10.1016/j.psyneuen.2021.105211

[123] Siebert AP, Ma Z, Grevet JD, et al. Structural and functional similarities of calcium homeostasis modulator 1 (CALHM1) ion channel with connexins, pannexins, and innexins. Journal of Biological Chemistry. 2013;**288**:6140-6153. DOI: 10.1074/jbc.M112.409789

[124] Hernández-Salinas R, Vielma AZ, Arismendi MN, et al. Boldine prevents renal alterations in diabetic rats. Journal Diabetes Research. 2013;**2013**:1-12. DOI: 10.1155/2013/593672

[125] Toro CA, Johnson K, Hansen J, et al. Boldine modulates glial transcription and functional recovery in a murine model of contusion spinal cord injury. Frontiers in Cellular Neuroscience. 2023;**17**:1-16. DOI: 10.3389/fncel.2023.1163436

[126] Li H, Guo A, Salgado M, et al. The connexin hemichannel inhibitor D4 produces rapid antidepressant-like effects in mice. Journal of Neuroinflammation. 2023;**20**:191. DOI: 10.1186/s12974-023-02873-z

[127] Cisterna BA, Vargas AA, Puebla C, et al. Active acetylcholine receptors prevent the atrophy of skeletal muscles and favor reinnervation. Nature Communications. 2020;**11**:1073. DOI: 10.1038/s41467-019-14063-8

[128] Guo A, Zhang H, Li H, et al. Inhibition of connexin hemichannels alleviates neuroinflammation and hyperexcitability in temporal lobe epilepsy. Proceedings of the National Academy of Sciences. 2022;**119**:1-12. DOI: 10.1073/pnas.2213162119

[129] Walrave L, Pierre A, Albertini G, et al. Inhibition of astroglial connexin43 hemichannels with TAT-Gap19 exerts anticonvulsant effects in rodents. Glia. 2018;**66**:1788-1804. DOI: 10.1002/glia.23341

[130] Chen B, Yang L, Chen J, et al. Inhibition of Connexin43 hemichannels with Gap19 protects cerebral ischemia/reperfusion injury via the JAK2/STAT3 pathway in mice. Brain Research Bulletin. 2019;**146**:124-135. DOI: 10.1016/j.brainresbull.2018.12.009

[131] Chen Y, Wang L, Zhang L, et al. Inhibition of connexin 43 hemichannels alleviates cerebral ischemia/reperfusion injury via the TLR4 signaling pathway. Frontiers in Cellular Neuroscience. 2018;**12**:1-15. DOI: 10.3389/fncel.2018.00372

[132] Dierks A, Vanucci-Bacqué C, Schäfer A-M, et al. The bioactive

phenolic agents diaryl ether CVB2-61 and diarylheptanoid CVB4-57 as connexin hemichannel blockers. Pharmaceuticals. 2022;**15**:1173. DOI: 10.3390/ph15101173

[133] Yang HW, Kho AR, Lee SH, et al. A phosphodiesterase 4 (PDE4) inhibitor, amlexanox, reduces neuroinflammation and neuronal death after pilocarpine-induced seizure. Neurotherapeutics. 2024;**21**:e00357. DOI: 10.1016/j.neurot.2024.e00357

[134] Agarwal S, Vyas P, Nirwan N, et al. Effect of lacosamide on neuroinflammation-mediated seizures comorbid with depression in C57BL/6 mice– Role of kynurenine pathway. Epilepsy and Behavior. 2021;**123**:108262. DOI: 10.1016/j.yebeh.2021.108262

[135] Mat Nor MN, Rupenthal ID, Green CR, et al. Connexin hemichannel block using orally delivered tonabersat improves outcomes in animal models of retinal disease. Neurotherapeutics. 2020;**17**:371-387. DOI: 10.1007/s13311-019-00786-5

[136] Kim Y, Griffin JM, Nor MNM, et al. Tonabersat prevents inflammatory damage in the central nervous system by blocking connexin43 hemichannels. Neurotherapeutics. 2017;**14**:1148-1165. DOI: 10.1007/s13311-017-0536-9

[137] Lyon H, Shome A, Rupenthal ID, et al. Tonabersat inhibits connexin43 hemichannel opening and inflammasome activation in an in vitro retinal epithelial cell model of diabetic retinopathy. International Journal of Molecular Sciences. 2021;**22**:1-12. DOI: 10.3390/ijms22010298

[138] NIH National Library of Medicine. Tonabersat Clinical Trials. ClinicalTrialsGov; 2025. Available from: https://www.clinicaltrials.gov/search?intr=Tonabersat [Accessed: May 13, 2025]

[139] Yi C, Ezan P, Fernández P, et al. Inhibition of glial hemichannels by boldine treatment reduces neuronal suffering in a murine model of Alzheimer's disease. Glia. 2017;**65**:1607-1625. DOI: 10.1002/glia.23182

[140] Cipriani A, Zhou X, Del Giovane C, et al. Comparative efficacy and tolerability of antidepressants for major depressive disorder in children and adolescents: A network meta-analysis. The Lancet. 2016;**388**:881-890. DOI: 10.1016/S0140-6736(16)30385-3

[141] Toth M. Epigenetic neuropharmacology: Drugs affecting the epigenome in the brain. Annual Review of Pharmacology and Toxicology. 2021;**2025**(25):6. DOI: 10.1146/annurev-pharmtox-030220

[142] Trerotola M, Relli V, Simeone P, et al. Epigenetic inheritance and the missing heritability. Human Genomics. 2015;**9**:-17. DOI: 10.1186/s40246-015-0041-3

[143] Yang R, Gautam A, Getnet D, et al. Epigenetic biotypes of post-traumatic stress disorder in war-zone exposed veteran and active duty males. Molecular Psychiatry. 2021;**26**:4300-4314. DOI: 10.1038/s41380-020-00966-2

[144] Yuan M, Yang B, Rothschild G, et al. Epigenetic regulation in major depression and other stress-related disorders: Molecular mechanisms, clinical relevance and therapeutic potential. Signal Transduction and Targeted Therapy. 2023;**8**:309. DOI: 10.1038/s41392-023-01519-z

[145] Schiele MA, Domschke K. Epigenetics at the crossroads between genes, environment and resilience in anxiety disorders. Genes, Brain and Behavior. 2018;**17**:1-15. DOI: 10.1111/gbb.12423

[146] Mychasiuk R, Muhammad A, Kolb B. Chronic stress induces persistent changes in global DNA methylation and gene expression in the medial prefrontal cortex, orbitofrontal cortex, and hippocampus. Neuroscience. 2016;**322**:489-499. DOI: 10.1016/j.neuroscience.2016.02.053

[147] Perisic T, Zimmermann N, Kirmeier T, et al. Valproate and amitriptyline exert common and divergent influences on global and gene promoter-specific chromatin modifications in rat primary astrocytes. Neuropsychopharmacology. 2010;**35**:792-805. DOI: 10.1038/npp.2009.188

[148] Zimmermann N, Zschocke J, Perisic T, et al. Antidepressants inhibit DNA methyltransferase 1 through reducing G9a levels. Biochemical Journal. 2012;**448**:93-102. DOI: 10.1042/BJ20120674

[149] Rapanelli M, Williams JB, Ma K, et al. Targeting histone demethylase LSD1 for treatment of deficits in autism mouse models. Molecular Psychiatry. 2022;**27**:3355-3366. DOI: 10.1038/s41380-022-01508-8

[150] Ookubo M, Kanai H, Aoki H, et al. Antidepressants and mood stabilizers effects on histone deacetylase expression in C57BL/6 mice: Brain region specific changes. Journal of Psychiatric Research. 2013;**47**:1204-1214. DOI: 10.1016/j.jpsychires.2013.05.028

[151] Belujon P, Grace AA. Dopamine system dysregulation in major depressive disorders. International Journal of Neuropsychopharmacology. 2017;**20**:1036-1046. DOI: 10.1093/ijnp/pyx056

[152] Su Y, Li H, Zhang W, et al. Connexin43 hemichannel blockade turns microglia neuroprotective and mitigates cognitive deficits in a mouse model of amyloidosis. Nature Communications. 2025;**16**:5621. DOI: 10.1038/s41467-025-60746-w